SMART Recovery™

4-POINT PROGRAM®
HANDBOOK

The SMART Recovery 4-Point Program® Handbook

4th edition
SMART Recovery®
7304 Mentor Avenue, Suite F
Mentor, OH 44060

Phone (440) 951-5357
Email information@smartrecovery.org
Web www.smartrecovery.org

4th Ed. Contributors: A. Tom Horvath, PhD; Peter J. Rubinas
Editor: Louisa Diodato
Publisher: SMART Recovery USA, Inc.
Copyright 2025, SMART Recovery International
ISBN: 978-1-7342388-7-7

Table of Contents

Welcome to SMART

This 4-Point Handbook is for those experiencing problems with substances like alcohol, opiates, tobacco, meth, and other drugs. It can also be used for activities that may become addictive like sexual activity, gaming, gambling, shopping, and eating. SMART is adaptable, too. It can help you change any behavior pattern that interferes with your life, job, or relationships.

Whoever you are, whatever you're going through, we're glad you're here. SMART is Self-Management and Recovery Training. It's an approach for anyone who wants to make a positive change in their life.

For family members and friends

Concerned family members and friends are welcome in the SMART community too. SMART is about self-empowerment, meaning each person controls their own choices. As partners, parents, children, siblings, spouses, and peers, you can't change your loved one's behavior. But you can learn how to manage your relationship, your emotional reactions, and your expectations. And you can learn to be a positive support instead of perpetuating stigma or creating unproductive pressure.

This handbook is specifically for individuals who want to change an addictive behavior, but it can help you understand your loved one's journey too. SMART's separate Family & Friends handbook and group meetings are more specifically tailored to your needs. You can find both on the SMART Recovery website.

Seek professional help if you need it

SMART isn't a substitute for professional help or treatment from a therapist, counselor, psychologist, or psychiatrist. It can, however, supplement any professional help or treatment you are receiving. And it has helped many people work toward positive change on their own.

You may be able to find a SMART-supportive mental health professional in your area on the SMART Recovery website.

Managing a crisis or withdrawal

SMART isn't an acute crisis service, even though you may be able to find a meeting to join right now. If you live in the United States or Canada, consider calling or texting 988 instead. The 988 Lifeline is a network of local crisis centers that provide free, confidential support to anyone in emotional distress (including those considering suicide) 24 hours a day.

If you're going through withdrawal, consider getting medical care. That could mean finding a doctor, emergency room, or urgent care center. If you feel unsafe getting there alone, have someone bring you. Withdrawal can be severe or fatal, and your safety is important.

What and who is SMART?

This handbook is published by SMART Recovery USA, a nonprofit affiliate of SMART Recovery International. While SMART partners with other organizations from time to time, we are not affiliated with any governmental agency, court, corrections facility, treatment center, political party, or religious group.

Most of our meetings are facilitated by trained volunteers, with some led by professionals. There's no fee to participate and no registration required unless specified in a meeting's listing on the SMART Recovery website.

SMART is funded in part by donations from participants and supporters along with local, state, and federal grants. We hope you consider giving back to SMART in line with the help you receive from it. Learn more about donating on the SMART Recovery website.

Visit the SMART Recovery website to read about our values, position statements, and what we expect of our volunteers.

Will SMART work for me?

While many people around the world find SMART helpful, there are no guarantees. What works for one person in one situation may not work for another. You don't need a formal diagnosis of a substance use disorder to benefit from SMART. And it doesn't matter whether you consider your issue mild, moderate, or severe. All that matters is that you want to make a change or are considering a change.

Scientists know which treatments work well, but they know less about how and why they work. Still, research shows that mutual support groups like SMART and professional treatment are effective. The most important features of the approaches like SMART that work are:

- Learning coping skills
- Learning how to live without the behavior you find problematic
- Connecting with others
- Giving back
- Increasing your self-confidence

Participants who stick with SMART tend to value these features in our approach:

- **Self-empowering:** You make your own choices.
- **Science-informed:** We keep up with developments in science.
- **Progress-oriented:** You decide what your goals are. Abstinence does not have to be one of them.
- **Holistic:** We focus on your whole life, not just the behavior you find problematic.
- **Nonexclusive:** You can combine SMART's approach with any other approaches that help you.

Therapeutic foundations

SMART's 4-Point Program was originally based on concepts from rational emotive behavior therapy (REBT). REBT was the first form of cognitive behavior therapy pioneered by Dr. Albert Ellis in the 1950s. REBT is based on the premise that how we think influences how we feel, and how we feel influences how we act. Thinking about a life event one way leads to certain feelings and actions. By reinterpreting that same event, we may be able to change the feelings that arise and the actions that follow. As the science of behavior change has advanced, we've added additional concepts to our approach from current therapeutic and behavioral approaches.

For many participants the fundamental tool in SMART is realizing that we can view ourselves, our situations, and our futures differently. As the philosopher Epictetus said centuries ago: "We are disturbed not by events but by our views about them."

Addictive behaviors often arise from hard-to-manage emotions. Hard-to-manage emotions often come from unhelpful thinking about a life event or interaction. We cover this idea more thoroughly in Chapter 5.

Multiple pathways

The process of change looks different for everyone. Although SMART works for many, we don't believe it's the only helpful path. We also don't ask you to use SMART exclusively.

Our participants are welcome to try other approaches instead of or alongside ours. Many combine SMART with:

- Other mutual support groups
- Prescribed medications
- Psychotherapy
- Residential treatment
- A recovery coach
- Living in a recovery residence, etc.

Our participants also pursue passions that support positive change. Some start exercising, changing their eating, volunteering in their communities (and for SMART), making new friends, planting gardens—you name it. There are as many pathways to change as there are individuals.

You are welcome to use SMART however it suits you best, and to come and go as you need. You're always welcome back.

Chapter 1
Starting SMART

SMART's 4-Point Program® consists of this handbook and associated mutual support meetings. Both consider the same four aspects of behavior change:

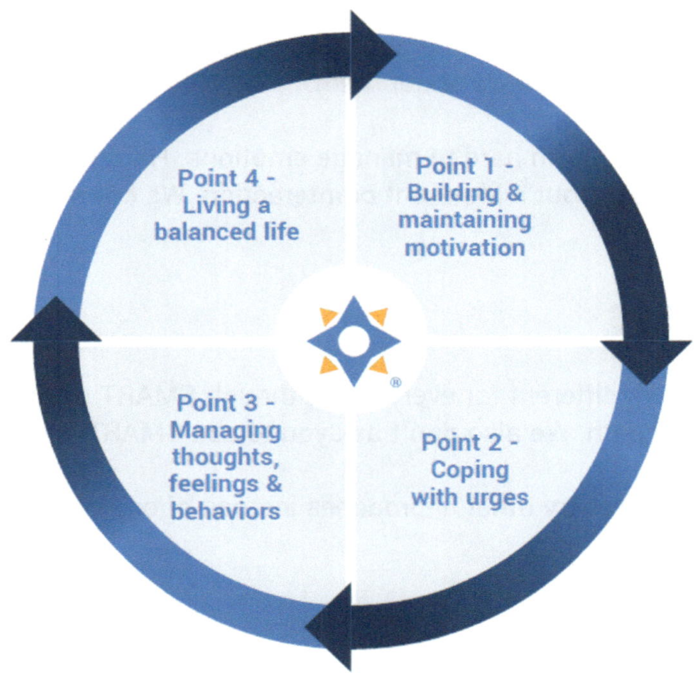

The points are groupings of ideas and tools for you to consider. You can focus on them in any order and at any time, you might shift your focus from one to another. It all depends on where you're at in your journey at that time. Like a compass, the points can help you stay on course.

How to use this handbook

For some, this handbook is a living record of their journey. We encourage you to write notes, questions, and responses as you go. You can download additional printable copies of some tools from the SMART Recovery website.

Using this handbook alone could be enough to create meaningful change for you. For many people, attending SMART meetings is an important support as they practice what they learn.

Meetings

Meetings are the heart of the SMART 4-Point approach. Interacting with others will help reinforce that you're not alone. The heartfelt words of peers who've walked a similar path can help build your confidence. At the same time, your experiences help others. You can look up meetings in your area on the SMART Recovery website.

Know that facilitator styles vary. Some meetings focus on a particular tool, while others are discussion based. Visit a few different meetings before you decide whether SMART is the right approach for you. You're welcome to start and stop attending as you need.

If you're debating between attending SMART meetings and seeking professional help, remember you can do both. And if you choose to tackle your journey without meetings, that's OK too.

What facilitators do

In SMART, the facilitator guides the meeting. You're welcome and encouraged to speak directly to your peers. Like the facilitator, you too can steer the conversation, provided you do so respectfully. For example, you might say to the facilitator: "I see you're moving forward with the planned topic for tonight. But could we return to what Sandra just told us about a binge over the weekend?" And then, directly to the peer: "Would you like to talk about what happened, or what led up to it? Or how you got out of it? I think it would be helpful to all of us."

The facilitator is free to overrule this idea, and your peer doesn't have to say more. But the group will appreciate your assertiveness. And your peer may appreciate you showing an interest.

Discussion

Facilitators can structure meetings in a variety of ways. Here are examples of what you may encounter in a SMART meeting:

- **Welcome and introductions**
- **Check-in.** Some meetings are almost entirely check-ins. Others, including large online meetings, may not have check-ins at all. During check-ins, each person speaks either around a circle or in the order they volunteer. There could be some discussion after each check-in.
- **Discussion.** The facilitator might have prepared a specific topic or Tool for this part of the meeting. Or a focus might flow naturally from what came up during check-in. Sometimes the facilitator will go around the circle. Other times there's an open discussion.
- **Checkout.** If someone shared something helpful for you, this is the time to thank them. Everyone benefits from thanks. You can also say what was most meaningful to you or share a fresh commitment to yourself. Other closing ideas are welcome too.

Please see our most current meeting guidelines on the SMART Recovery website. Specific information about individual meetings may also appear in the meeting's listing on the website.

Off-topic subjects

In our experience, the following topics tend to become debates. They distract rather than help anyone make positive change. For that reason, facilitators will typically redirect conversations away from:

- Whether addiction is a disease
- Whether you need the help of a "higher power" to change
- Whether it's better for everyone to abstain from or moderate a specific behavior
- What's "wrong" with any other approaches to change

You're welcome to have a viewpoint on any or all of these topics. And it's also OK to briefly state your beliefs when it's relevant. For example:

- "Coming to SMART meetings and going to church have been the foundation of how I've quit using."
- "I don't believe in a higher power, so I've spent a lot of my time defining what my values and beliefs are."
- "I've decided abstinence is the best thing for me. I admire the people here who are successfully moderating. I've tried that route enough. Abstinence is the best route for me."
- "I tried AA for a while. I liked the people, but I didn't want to label myself as an alcoholic."

The facilitator may redirect the conversation at any time if it seems to be going in an unhelpful direction.

Civility and non-judgment

SMART meetings should be civil at a minimum. There's no criticism, unwanted advice, teasing, or rude comments, and certainly no raised voices. An atmosphere of non-judgment is even better.

Sometimes we discuss intense, life-threatening experiences. Nonjudgment doesn't mean we support any of the unhealthy behavior we talk about. Instead, it means we trust that our peers are making the best decisions they can in each situation. Those situations can include intense urges, strong emotions, and a belief that we need relief right away.

Remember that participants come to SMART in all stages of their journey. Some have maintained chosen patterns of behavior for years, while others are just now considering change. Meetings are valuable because the participants discuss their urges, emotions, and beliefs, which can be very private. It doesn't feel safe to share them when you expect to be criticized. Besides, we're all on a journey of change. If we didn't see or suspect the harm in our own behavior, we wouldn't be here. We don't need someone else to point it out.

Sometimes the most valuable meetings focus on someone's return to old behaviors. It's not uncommon for people to return to their old behaviors before succeeding in establishing a new chosen pattern of behavior. It's a normal part of the process, so it's crucial we discuss these episodes freely. It can help each of us learn to prevent or reduce future returns to old behaviors.

Getting the most from meetings

- Be willing to learn. New ideas, tools, and interpretations are valuable. Once you're a regular in a particular meeting, you might start taking notes about helpful ideas you hear.
- Be open and honest. It can be hard, but it's a crucial part of learning. Consider planning what you'll say about yourself ahead of time to make it easier.
- Prepare when you can. Read a part of the handbook, watch videos, or listen to podcasts. You'll be able to bring ideas to others in the meeting. (It also means you're thinking about change even when you're not in a meeting.)

- Balance speaking and listening. In some meetings, you can focus on listening. In others, your concerns may be the focus of the discussion for a while. Both are normal. Do what makes sense for that meeting.
- Look at the big picture. Exercising more, changing your eating, sleeping well, and connecting with others may all be a part of your journey. Focus on these when you're not in meetings and talk about them when you attend.

Meeting FAQs

Are SMART meetings confidential?

Yes. Everyone is expected to keep who attended and what was said private.

How do I attend a meeting?

Just show up unless a meeting listing on the SMART Recovery website states otherwise. The website listing contains essential information about each meeting.

When/where do meetings occur?

Visit the SMART Recovery website for a full list of meetings. If you're interested in meetings for a specific audience, you'll find those marked as such.

How long do meetings last?

Meetings typically last 60 or 90 minutes.

If I attend, what am I required to do?

It's totally up to you. You can speak when a facilitator opens the discussion to you, or you can pass. You don't have to give your name or any other personal information. If you're in an online meeting, you don't have to have your camera on.

Who are the facilitators?

Typically they're trained volunteers who are also SMART participants. Some may be led by professionals. Anyone is welcome to facilitate meetings, regardless of their history with addictive behaviors. It may be a family member who's been inspired to bring SMART to their community.

Why would SMART have facilitators who haven't experienced addictive behavior?

SMART facilitators keep the discussion on track. The expertise about change comes from other participants and SMART's publications. Experienced facilitators bring a lot to the group, even without a personal history of addictive behavior.

Can my attendance be verified?

If you need to provide verification of attendance to someone else, many SMART meetings can provide them. See the individual meeting listings on the SMART website for details.

Is there a charge to attend meetings?

SMART meetings are always free to attend. Donations are requested to help cover meeting costs and other expenses, but you're not required to contribute. Organizations that host private meetings for their clients may not charge extra for their clients to participate in SMART meetings.

Can students, professionals in training, professionals, or others interested in learning about SMART attend?

Yes. Meetings are open to the public unless the website listing states otherwise.

Are there specific meetings for newcomers?

Newcomers are welcome in all meetings. It's helpful to let others know you're new at check-in. Questions are welcome before, during, and after meetings.

Do I need to attend meetings for the rest of my life?

No. But if you want to, you can. And you can always drop by occasionally when you want to reconnect.

How does it work to have so many different people and experiences in one meeting?

We're all eager to learn from one another. Recognizing the experiences we share despite our differences is often an important source of motivation.

Becoming a facilitator

Most facilitators say that facilitating is one of the most helpful things they did for themselves and their change journey. If and when you're ready, ask a facilitator you know about the process. You might ask them to mentor you.

You can ease into facilitating by leading certain parts of the meeting with your mentor's guidance. For example:

- Read the welcome
- Keep the meeting running on time
- Lead check-in

Ideally, facilitators promote discussion more than they "teach" tools. But as you learn to facilitate, you'll learn much more about the tools, too. Most important: Facilitating is a huge contribution to your community. If you're looking for a way to help others, this is a great option.

SMART's tools

Think of the activities throughout this handbook as tools. Physical tools help people extend or improve their abilities. The tools in SMART are mental tools, but they work much the same way. Each section and its tools are designed to help you learn and remember. Know that SMART didn't invent the tools you find here. We adapted them from proven theories.

The outcomes from using tools vary. You can use a hammer to drive nails or smash holes in a wall. The cost benefit analysis in Section 3 could be used to conclude that the long-term costs of your behavior exceed the short-term benefits. Or, with the same set of facts you, you could mislead yourself to conclude "I don't have a problem."

Discussions in meetings are one way to learn about tools. You may not fully understand the depth of a tool until you've discussed it in a meeting. You can observe how others are practicing and learning them. Other participants can also learn from you.

Some tools you might return to over and over. Others you might not use at all. They're just suggestions. You're also welcome to mention tools or activities from outside SMART. Your peers will benefit from hearing about what has worked for you.

Summary

- SMART is an approach for anyone struggling with any addictive behavior.
- Meetings are a great way to connect with others. They're also a place to practice what you learn in this handbook.

Chapter 2
First steps

Understanding addictive behaviors

People can enjoy or benefit from many substances and activities without problems. But anything can start causing problems if it becomes too big a part of our lives. We call any substance or activity that has become problematic an addictive behavior.

You might choose to describe your behaviors as addictive when they:

- Become a strong habitual pattern
- Become stronger each time you do them
- Involve short-term rewards or immediate satisfaction, but lead to longer-term costs, like damaged relationships or financial problems
- Start to crowd out other sources of satisfaction
- Lead you to violate your values

Only you can decide when your behavior has become problematic enough that you want to address it. SMART's tools can help.

Is addiction a disease?

There's debate among medical and behavioral health professionals around whether addiction is accurately described as a disease. Thankfully, it doesn't really matter in SMART. Our approach can help you regardless of whether you believe addiction is a disease or not. That's because we focus on what you can control–changing your behavior in the ways that work best for you.

Systems 1 and 2 thinking: Moving beyond Immediate satisfaction to intentional choice

The human brain is complex. We may feel that we are making conscious decisions all day long. However, most of our behaviors happen automatically in response to cues or triggers in our environment. We see a red light, and we stop. When that light turns green, we go. We don't reprocess what red lights and green lights mean each time we encounter them. This is an amazing gift when what we learn to do automatically is helpful!

The same thing happens as we learn how to navigate strong emotions in our lives. If an experience creates strong feelings of anxiety or sadness, your brain notices activities that help resolve them quickly. Similarly, your brain notices behaviors that efficiently lead to feelings of joy or pleasure. Over time, your brain builds a whole library of automatic responses to the world that you aren't even aware of.

One helpful way cognitive scientists describe this is by differentiating between System 1 and System 2 thinking. System 1 thinking is automatic, effortless thinking that leads to strong habits, including addictive behaviors. System 2 thinking is slow, mindful, and requires much more effort.

The tools in SMART are designed to help you engage in System 2 thinking. You'll learn to slow down and become aware of your patterns of behavior. What triggers are you experiencing? What urges or cravings can you notice earlier? How can you interrupt an automatic response and replace it with a healthier one?

Characteristics of System 1 and System 2 Thinking	
System 1 thinking	**System 2 thinking**
Fast Automatic Spontaneous Effortless Intuitive Reflexive Impulsive	Slow Methodical Intentional Effortful Deliberate Conscious Mindful

Immediate satisfaction often has a stronger pull than healthier, delayed rewards. Every time we satisfy an urge with an automatic response, we strengthen a pattern of immediate satisfaction: You felt better last time you did this, so it's a good idea. The next urge comes more quickly and more forcefully.

Know this is a cycle you can escape. You're not doomed to repeat it forever. Keep hope and look for your exit. Millions of people have done it and moved on to more satisfying lives. It happens every day.

How to gain independence from an addictive behavior

As simplistic as it may sound, change can start by slowing down your thinking and becoming more aware of it. The first step is becoming aware of your urges. Then you can practice not responding immediately to them. In doing so, the urges may become less intense and occur less frequently. Slowly, the triggers that created them will lose their associations. The road will narrow, and you'll find you can manage it better. One key is learning to tolerate short-term discomfort. Urges often don't feel good, but they'll only last for seconds to minutes. (More on this in Chapter 3.) Eventually, they'll fade, and you'll more easily be able to control your next actions. That's you, retraining your brain.

For some, it only takes a few days or weeks to feel the difference. The short-term discomfort you feel starts paying off in the form of a healthier life. And that's when the addictive behavior starts losing its grip on you. You'll see your addictive behavior as a choice, not an inevitable reaction to discomfort. And once it's a choice, it's yours to make.

How SMART can help

Your path to positive change can be a realistic and self-directed journey. SMART can help you:

- Identify and understand the triggers that lead to your cravings and urges
- Realize that triggers don't have to result in addictive behavior
- Cope with your urges and make better decisions
- Stay motivated and focused, even when a situation seems overwhelming
- Change how you think about the events in your life

Recovery: A term you may choose to use

The term recovery may not mean much to you if the change you're looking for is small, or if you are not planning to abstain from anything. Or it might mean a lot to you. Let's talk about what recovery might be. It may not be as obvious as you assume.

SAMHSA (the Substance Abuse and Mental Health Services Administration) defines recovery as:

> **a process of change through which individuals improve their health and wellness, live a self-directed life, and strive to reach their full potential**

Notice how broad that definition is. It's not only about changing the behavior that's causing problems in your life. In fact, it doesn't mention that at all. It's about your wellness, your empowerment, and your potential. When we use the term "recovery" in this handbook, that's what we mean. You don't need to use it if it doesn't feel right to you. You may prefer "change" or "process of change," another term, or no term at all.

What recovery could look like for you

The process of change is different for everyone. Yours might involve changing negative thinking patterns. You might abstain from certain behaviors. You might commit to trying new activities that challenge you or making more time for your loved ones.

If you focus only on reducing or resolving an addictive behavior, you leave a gap behind. To create a more balanced life, many replace addictive behaviors with healthier activities. That's Chapter 6. But again: The process of change is a personal journey. It's what you make it and can be whatever you want it to be.

The words you use matter

There's a lot of stigma around addictive behaviors. Maybe you've been called names or been told you're weak or different from other people. Maybe you've been given an ultimatum or told you'll never change. You may have noticed: This type of input is typically not helpful!

That's because this kind of talk can make your situation feel hopeless. There's a big difference between "a drunk" and "someone who struggles with drinking." If you let your behavior determine your identity, it can feel harder to change. And if you think "I'll never be able to change this," then why bother trying?

Hopelessness can make addictive behaviors stronger and that's why we don't use labels in SMART. You might consider not applying labels to yourself unless it helps motivate you. If others apply them to you, respectfully correct them when you can.

Changing the dialogue

Like any long journey, the process of change usually starts with small steps. Changing behavior takes time and effort, trial and error. Instead of what you might have told yourself in the past, try:

- I can choose not to act on addictive urges anymore.
- I'm more than the behaviors I want to change.
- I'm in control of my choices and actions.

Those words may help you feel more confident, especially at the beginning of your journey. If you believe you'll overcome your addictive behaviors, you probably will. If one of SMART's strategies or activities doesn't work for you, try a different one until you find what makes you successful. Change is possible. Urges fade away. Making healthy choices gets easier. Your addictive behavior becomes a thing of your past. You find meaning and enjoyment in your new life.

Abstinence, moderation, and harm/risk reduction

The idea of abstinence can be intimidating or even distasteful as you begin your journey. You're welcome at SMART meetings regardless of whether you want to try abstinence or not.

For substance use, abstinence means that you stop drinking or using. It also applies to some compulsive behaviors, like gambling, because you don't need to gamble to survive. It's harder to abstain from behaviors like eating, shopping, and sex. These are a normal part of life. Someone who struggles with eating behaviors, for example, still needs to eat.

Even though SMART doesn't require abstinence, you might consider abstinence for yourself because:

- Even approaches aimed at controlled use or moderation usually recommend stopping completely at first. It can be an effective way to start, even if moderation is your long-term goal.

- It may be easier to abstain than moderate addictive behavior, because it's obvious when you drift. Moderating means setting limits and monitoring them, analyzing every choice. Even someone who's committed to change can find their behavior inching back toward old patterns.
- Since it's simpler, you can focus on other aspects of the change process. What goals do you have for yourself? What else do you love to do?

You might decide to choose abstinence as a goal because:

- It's simple. There's no counting, no precise decisions, and it applies in all situations.
- You'll recognize positive changes and improve your confidence more quickly.
- Continued addictive behavior, even in smaller amounts, could aggravate medical, psychological, or psychiatric conditions.
- Even moderate substance use could interfere with prescribed medications. (And sometimes the interactions are dangerous.)
- You are pregnant or plan to become pregnant.
- You're under social pressure to abstain—from family, friends, an employer, or a court.
- Your personal or family history might put you at risk of depression or violence.

Longer term, abstinence might help you understand how you feel without a substance or behavior. And better self-understanding can provide insight on how you got where you are and where you want to go.

Even if you continue your current level of addictive behavior, there are changes you can make to reduce your harm or risk of harm, as well as the risk of harm to others. For instance, if you drink, you can choose not to drive. If you inject drugs, you can choose to test the drugs and use clean needles. A SMART meeting is a good place to talk about how you might keep yourself and others safer.

It's your choice to make

In a self-empowering approach like SMART, you choose your own goals. You might have different goals for different substances or activities. You might abstain, moderate, or reduce risk. You can change your goals at any time. Whatever you choose, it's not a commitment to be perfect. Getting off track is a normal part of the process for many people. We are here to help you stay on track or get back on track when needed.

Recognize the seriousness of physical dependence

If you've used a substance heavily for a long time, **talk to a doctor, mental health professional, or call 988 before you stop**. This includes alcohol. "Going cold turkey" (abstaining suddenly and completely) can be dangerous or even life-threatening.

Stages of change

Changing a long-standing behavior probably won't be simple. Many people move in and out of different stages of change until they achieve a new normal. Even then, some still return occasionally to old patterns of behavior.

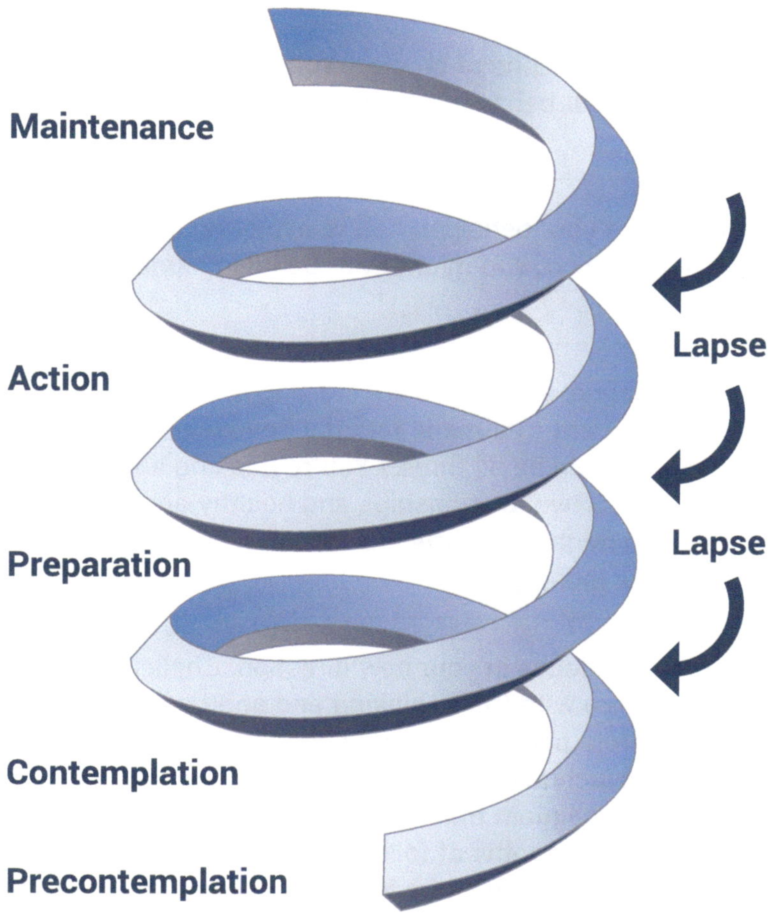

Model developed by James Prochaska and Carlo DiClemente in the 1970s.

As you read the descriptions of each stage below, consider which stage you're in today. Tomorrow might be different. For example: Today you might be in Preparation, because you're committed to change. But maybe tomorrow you have doubts, so you're back in Contemplation. You could even bounce between the stages over the course of a day. Knowing where you are isn't about congratulating yourself one day or chastising yourself the next. It's about understanding what you need in the present moment.

Precontemplation	You are not interested in change. Maybe you don't see a problem with your behavior. Your partner, employer, family, or a court might insist you get help from a group like SMART. But you might not agree that you have an addictive behavior. For the most part, you think external forces are responsible for your behavior. You might blame genetics, your family, society, or the legal system. You might think change is impossible.
Contemplation	You're weighing the pros and cons of change. You might have mixed feelings about changing your behavior. You like some things about it, but not others.
Preparation	You've decided to change your behavior. You're exploring options and alternatives to make it happen. You might even be taking small steps toward change already.
Action	You're committed to change, and others are starting to see it. Maybe you've signed up for inpatient treatment, found a counselor, or joined a mutual-help group. (It could be all three.) You're thinking about the future, not the past. Supportive relationships and healthy activities are important here. Yes, you might be a little anxious—but you accept that discomfort as part of the journey.
Maintenance	You're building more confidence in your new direction. Challenges remain, and you meet them with fresh thinking and approaches. You're getting support from people you trust and focusing on healthy activities. You've achieved a new normal and are committed to the behaviors that will maintain that new normal. Professionals supporting you may use six months of following a new pattern of behavior as a benchmark for being in the Maintenance stage.
Lapses and relapses	You may or may not experience these, but they're common at any stage. They don't mean you have to start all over. In a lapse or relapse, you learn what worked or didn't. They can be brief, especially if you don't dwell on them. Many terms are used to describe these experiences, and some people don't find the terms "lapse" and "relapse" helpful. Choose the language that works best for you. Lapses and relapses will be discussed further in Chapter 5.

Start practicing!

Ready to start working on changes instead of just reading about them? Find a full listing of this handbook's tools on page 87. For more copies of select tools, see page 89.

We'll start off by introducing two activities that you might find helpful throughout your journey.

Tool 2.1: Journaling

Keeping a journal can be helpful in every stage of change. It's a record of your progress, setbacks, and accomplishments. It's a private place to document your experiences and emotions as they happen.

There are no rules in journaling. Use a favorite pen and notebook, save a file on your computer, or use a phone app. Write every day or only when you urgently need to think something through. Ditch lined paper if you like and draw or doodle. Keep your journal forever or throw it away. It's completely up to you.

Your journal is a place to:

- Congratulate yourself on an accomplishment
- Keep daily notes about thoughts, feelings, and activities
- Think through different parts of a complicated problem
- Plan activities or short-term goals
- Record what's helping you or holding you back
- Chart your progress

In journaling, you write about what is most important to you to understand it better. With practice, journaling can help you regulate your emotions more effectively.

Your journal is your space, and you can choose to share or keep it private. Some people are afraid to journal because someone else might read it. If that's you, tell others you live with that your journal is off limits. If you can't be that direct, consider keeping your journal with you or hiding it somewhere secure.

TIP

Find SMART tools for each stage of change in the quick reference guide on page 87.

Tool 2.2: Practice self-compassion

Self-compassion is a practice that can help address feelings of sadness or hopelessness. These feelings often arise when addressing an addictive behavior. One model of self-compassion defines it as a practice comprised of these three things:

- Being kind to yourself rather than judging yourself
- Recognizing that what you struggle with is something that you have in common with other humans
- Practicing mindfulness rather than over-identifying with your thoughts and emotions.

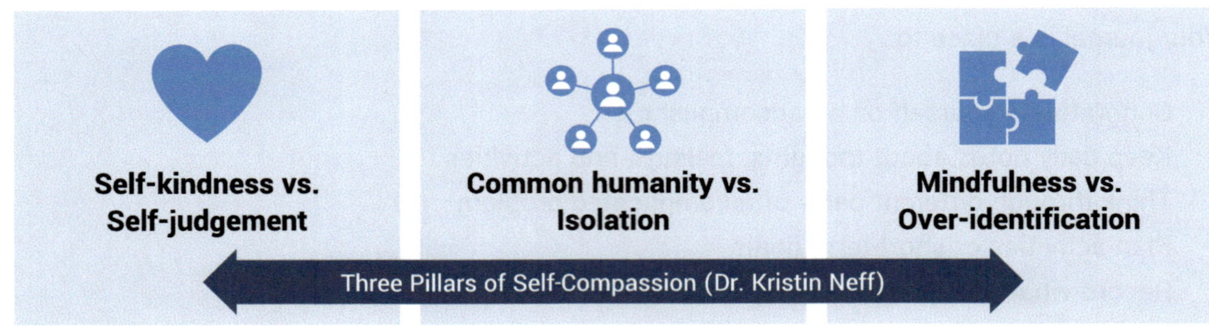

How can you practice these three things in your life? Jot some ideas down below. Pick one at a time to practice until they become habitual. With practice, you may find that self-compassion arises more quickly and with less effort, helping you stay present in each moment and reducing your stress.

Self-kindness practices	Common humanity practice	Mindfulness practice
Ex: Ask myself if that's how I would talk to a friend in this situation, stop calling myself names	Ex: Attend mutual support group meetings, volunteer	Ex: Daily meditation; notice the birds I hear on a walk

Chapter Summary

- Any initially enjoyable behavior can become addictive when it unbalances our lives. Addictive behaviors threaten our relationships, careers, freedom, and independence.
- SMART tools are designed to help you engage in Systems 2 thinking, moving from immediate satisfaction to intentional choice.
- You don't have to commit to abstinence now or ever, but there are reasons you might consider it.
- Keeping a journal and practicing self-compassion and mindfulness can be helpful.
- You're welcome in SMART regardless of what stage of change you're in or what your goals are.

Chapter 3
Point 1: Building and maintaining motivation

You probably already have some motivation to change. Otherwise, you wouldn't be reading this handbook. Maybe you're riding the emotional wave of a recent crisis. Maybe you're tired of criticism. Maybe a loved one or court requires you to show an effort. Whatever brought you here, you could have said no, and you didn't. What matters now is whether and how you nurture that motivation once the initial motivation fades.

Consider a past New Year's resolution. How long did it last? Most people struggle to stick with their goals, regardless of how small they are. Good intentions aren't enough. Neither is talking about what we want to achieve or trying to wish it into happening. What matters is building and maintaining genuine and personally meaningful motivation to continue taking positive steps forward.

This chapter will help you identify what motivates you and keeps you invested. Like everything else in SMART, this work is about self-empowerment. You decide what matters to you and what goals you set for your future.

Tool 3.1: Cost-benefit analysis

You get something out of the behavior you're thinking about changing. Otherwise, you wouldn't have engaged in it. Consciously or otherwise, at some point you decided the benefits outweighed the costs. Do they now?

It's normal to both want to change and not want to change. It's also difficult to hold the short- and long-term benefits and costs of a behavior in one's awareness at the same time. This tool can help with these challenges.

Write your benefits and costs in the boxes below. See page 27 for some questions to get you started.

The behavior I'm analyzing:

Today's date:

When I do this behavior

Benefits (rewards or advantages)	**Costs (risks and disadvantages)**
Ex: I feel more alert, I don't feel pain, I feel more attractive	Ex: Hangovers, losing my partner's trust*, hard to pay my bills on time

When I don't do this behavior

Benefits (rewards or advantages)	**Costs (risks and disadvantages)**
Ex: Save money*, do better at work	Ex: Feel stressed, body aches

After you make your lists, star the long-term benefits and costs. Where are you sacrificing your future goals for immediate satisfaction in the present?

More copies on page 89

Common costs and benefits for addictive behavior

To identify benefits in your behavior, ask yourself:

- What pleasures or advantages does it bring to my life?
- What emotions, feelings, or moods does it help me moderate? (Frustration, anger, fear, boredom, depression, anxiety, loneliness, stress?)
- How does it help me cope?
- What positive feelings, moods, or situations does it make better?
- What things does it help, or at least help me do better?
- Does it help me avoid reality or escape?
- Does it ease or reduce physical or emotional pain?
- Does it help me socialize and fit in?
- Do I need it to seem more fun, charming, interesting, or confident?
- Does it help me feel normal?

To identify costs of your behavior, ask yourself:

- What do I dislike about it?
- How is it harming me (physically, socially, mentally)?
- What will my life be like if I continue what I'm doing?
- How much time have I lost to it? How much time do I spend on it?
- Do I lie to hide my addictive behavior?
- How do I feel after the effects wear off?
- Does using affect my energy, stamina, or concentration?
- How much money have I spent on it?
- What legal problems does it create for me?
- What does it do to my relationships?
- How does it affect my work performance?
- What effects does it have on my self-respect and self-confidence?

To identify the rewards of stopping your behavior, ask yourself:

- How will stopping affect my health?
- How will it affect my relationships with the ones I love?
- How will stopping affect my job?
- How much money can I save?
- What will stopping do to my self-respect and self-confidence?
- Will stopping affect my ability to deal with my problems?
- What will I do with the time I don't spend on addictive behavior?
- What goals have I abandoned that I could accomplish?

To identify the costs of stopping your behavior:

- What will I miss about it?
- What issues in my life will I need a new solution for?
- What thoughts and emotions will I have to learn to accept/cope with?
- What do I like about my life that will change when I stop?

Tool 3.2: Define your values (hierarchy of values)

We all have values in life. And although they underpin all our feelings and decisions, we rarely think about them explicitly. Examining them and writing them down can help you focus on what matters most.

Start by jotting down as many of your values as you can—anything that you think matters to you. There are no right or wrong answers. Some examples: financial independence, my family, honesty, being happy, the environment, travel, solitude, or my health.

Next, go back and circle the big ones, or group your notes into themes. Ultimately, try to narrow your list to your top five.

My values
1.
2.
3.
4.
5.

What actions align with your values?

Now, look over your list. For most people, the behavior they want to change isn't a value. Yet it may have made itself a priority in your life. Where does your behavior conflict with your value system?

Notes:

Tool 3.3: Five questions about getting what I want

Sometimes it's hard to see what you could do differently to achieve your goals. Your goal in this exercise may be to reduce or resolve an addictive behavior, or it may be something broader.

1. What do I want for my future?

Examples: To get my degree, to be a good parent, to be financially independent

2. What am I doing to achieve that now?

Ex: Bookmarked ideas, talked to a friend, started an application

3. How do I feel about what I'm doing now?

Ex: Dissatisfied, stuck, guilty, stressed, disconnected

4. What could I do differently to help me get what I want?

5. How would changing what I do or getting what I want make me feel?

Compare your feelings about what you're doing (2) with how you'd feel if you changed your approach (5). Could the difference between the two motivate you? Could the activities in (4) help take the place of your addictive behavior? And if so—how much more quickly might you reach your goal in (1)?

Tool 3.4: Create a change plan

You're getting clearer about what you want for your future. Now you need a plan. Use this worksheet to identify steps you can take toward the future you envision. Consider who can help you get there. Remember that strategies are just ideas. If your first (or hundredth) plan doesn't work, try a new one.

My change plan	**Date:**
Changes I want to make: (Ex: Avoid bars/clubs, sleep better, abstain within 1 week)	
How important are these changes to me? (Rate from 1-10.)	
How confident am I that I can make these changes? (Rate from 1-10.)	
The most important reasons I want to make this change is: Ex: I want to keep my job, I want my kids back, I'm concerned about my health	
The steps I plan to take are: Ex: Attend SMART meetings, plan healthy meals each week, make a doctor's appointment	
Who can help me and how:	
Person	**Kind of help**
Ex: Friend	Share healthy recipes
I'll know my plan is working when: Ex: I can afford my own apartment, I'm always on time to work, I can have a normal conversation with my mom	
Some things that could interfere with my plan are: Ex: Having no plans on a weekend night, holiday season parties, last-minute changes to work schedule	
I'll check in with myself on this change plan on (date):	
Consider marking this date on your calendar, so you don't forget. If your plan isn't working out, edit it or start fresh and try again. More copies on page 89	

Hula hoop

Imagine you're standing inside a hula hoop. (Everyone else is standing inside their own hoop, too.) This visual can help remind you that what you can control is all inside your hula hoop. Everything outside of it is probably outside your control.

We spend an incredible amount of time and energy on things outside our hoop. Then, we get frustrated for failing to do what was impossible in the first place.

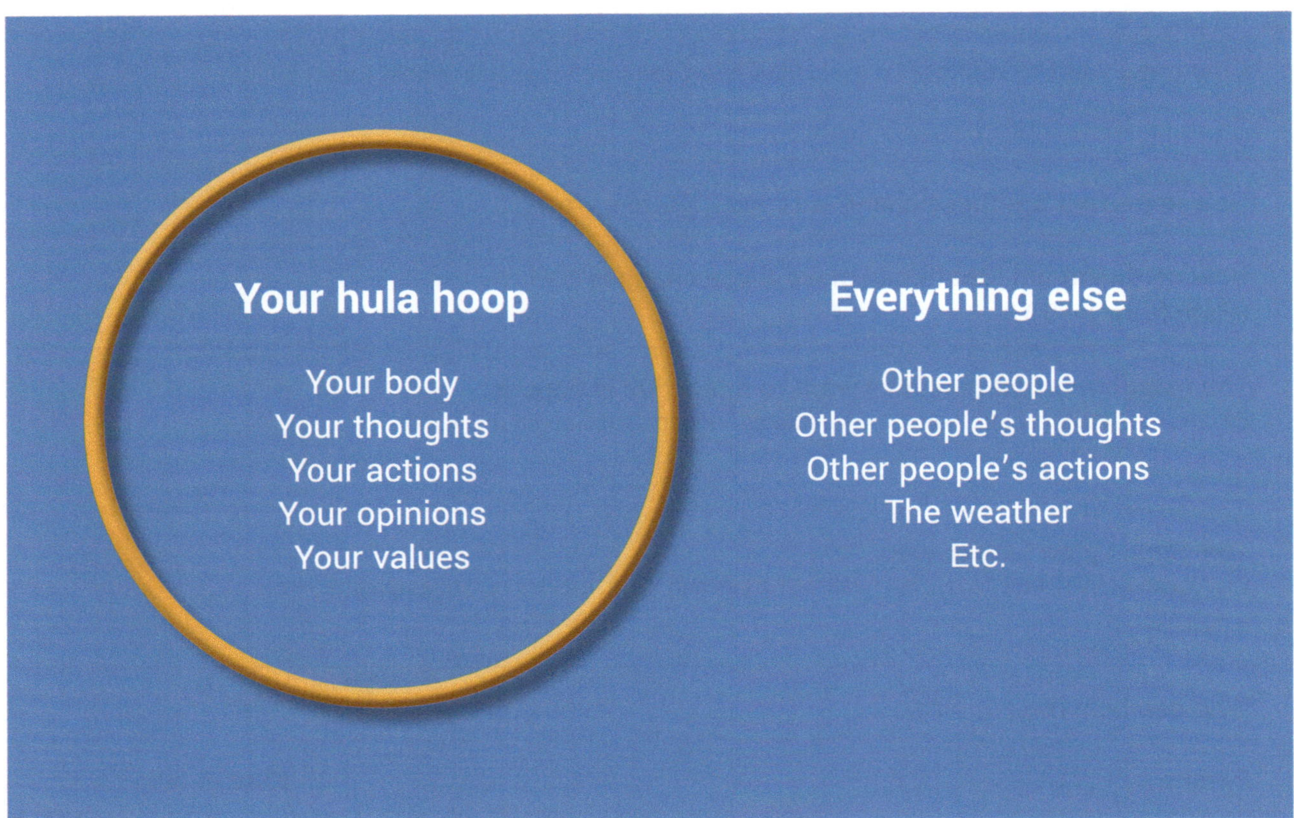

This may sound simple. But start sorting some things that frustrate you. How often are you in someone else's hula hoop? Are they in yours? Can you hula two hoops? (Maybe—but certainly not if the second hoop is around another person!)

Reflection and next steps

We hope the activities in this chapter have helped you to generate insights and have started to help you get a better idea of what you want your life to look like in the future.

Keep the tools you completed in this chapter handy. When you feel yourself being drawn to old behavior patterns, read them over again. You may find them especially useful as you learn to cope with urges—our next chapter.

Chapter Summary

- You learned that sustained motivation is the key to behavior change.
- You explored your own motivation in four ways:
  - –You weighed the costs and benefits of the behavior you may want to change.
  - –You identified your values.
  - –You envisioned your future consistent with those values
  - –You created a plan for change.
- Refer to your worksheets from this chapter any time you need to remotivate yourself.

Chapter 4
Point 2: Coping with urges

In Chapter 3, you explored tools about how to build your motivation. In this chapter, we'll explore how to deal with urges that might challenge your motivation. By "urges," we mean the social, mental, and emotional experience of wanting something. We're not talking about physical dependence or withdrawal symptoms.

Urges vs. withdrawal

How do I know what's an urge and what's a withdrawal symptom?
Individuals experiencing physical withdrawal from alcohol or another drug might experience the following symptoms:

- Nausea, vomiting, diarrhea
- Shaky hands
- Excessive sweating or rapid pulse
- Anxiety
- Agitation
- Physical sensations in the skin (itching, burning, numbness, etc).
- Auditory disturbances (sounds seem very loud or frightening, auditory hallucinations, etc.)
- Visual disturbances (light seems too bright, visual hallucinations, etc.)
- Headache
- Loss of orientation (who am I? where am I? what day is it?)
- Difficult sleeping, vivid unpleasant dreams, nightmares
- Seizures
- Pupils larger than normal
- Aches, physical discomfort, unable to sit still
- Runny nose, tears streaming down cheeks
- Yawning
- Depressed mood and activity
- Fever
- Excessive fatigue and sleepiness

What do I do if I'm experiencing withdrawal symptoms?

If you experience any of the withdrawal symptoms above, or other symptoms not on the list shortly after changing your use of alcohol or other drugs, consult with a medical professional immediately. If you are unsure whether you might experience withdrawal symptoms when stopping or reducing a behavior, err on the side of consulting with medical professionals in advance.

Learning to cope with urges is critical to making progress to reduce your addictive behavior. The feelings can be intense, and you're probably used to acting on them. It can be difficult, but it isn't always. Some people say they have no urges after deciding to quit. Others say they have urges later in their journey.

It helps to understand what urges are and why they happen. When you do, you can use them to learn tools to cope with them. Urges can be uncomfortable, but you can manage them. And for most, they eventually go away almost entirely or altogether.

Scratching an itch

If you've ever had a rash from something like poison oak or poison ivy, you know urges. The itch is intense. It can seem like the only relief is a long, hard scratch. And, yes, that feels satisfying in the short term. But it comes with consequences: The rash is slower healing, it scars, and it might get infected.

Similarly, you may feel like the only way to stop an urge is to give in. For rashes, there are anti-itch creams and oatmeal baths. And for addictive behaviors, there are healthy ways of coping. We'll work through some of them in this chapter.

Changing your understanding

First, let's debunk some common myths about urges. For some people, this alone can make urges easier to manage or prevent them completely.

Here are some opposing beliefs about urges that may help you understand them:

Myth	Fact
My urges are unbearable.	Urges won't kill you or make you crazy. They're uncomfortable, and you can learn to bear them. Telling yourself you can't is self-defeating.
Urges only stop when I give in.	Urges usually last for seconds or minutes, sometimes longer at the beginning. That's because eventually, your body adjusts. When you walk into a room with a strong smell, you notice it at first, and then it fades. That's the same effect you'll experience with urges.
My urges make me act on them.	Engaging in a behavior is always a choice, even when it feels like it isn't. You can choose to act on the urge, or you can ride it out.
Urges are a sign that my situation is not improving or getting worse.	Urges are a normal part of change. They might be strong early and then weaken, or weak early and then stronger. Both are normal.
Giving in to an urge isn't harmful.	Giving in reinforces the behavior pattern you want to change. The next urge usually comes stronger and faster than the last. Even a small allowance or dose still reinforces the pattern. And like scratching the rash, it can still be harmful and slow your healing time.
I need to get rid of urges.	Again, urges are normal. Addictive behaviors change your brain in ways that make urges feel powerful. You can't force them out of existence, but you can control how you respond. And that eventually weakens them.
I am self-destructive or I wouldn't do self-destructive things.	We're all human and we do unexplainable things sometimes.
I engage with my addictive behavior because I like to.	That might have been true in the beginning. It's probably more complicated than that now. You might also be ignoring the benefits of changing your behavior because you think it'll be too hard.

Urges aren't forever

Sticking with your change plan isn't signing up for a lifetime of discomfort. For most people, the first three months are hardest. After that, fewer people return to their old patterns of behavior.

The tools that follow will give you an advantage against urges. Combined with your motivation from Point 1, you really can cope with urges. Remember: It takes time and practice to replace old thoughts and behaviors with new ones. Don't expect urges to end immediately, don't expect to be perfect, and don't give up.

Triggers

Triggers are the things that lead to urges. Your brain has learned to associate them with addictive behaviors. They can be thoughts, emotions, activities, sights, sounds, sensations, tastes, smells, or a time of day, week, or year.

Each of us has our own triggers. Some are common across those with similar addictive behaviors. For example, someone who uses cocaine might be triggered by powders or tin foil. For someone who smokes, it might be meals, coffee, or alcohol. For someone who gambles, sports or store scratch-off cards could be a trigger. The great news is that triggers aren't unpredictable once you identify them. Your brain learned an association once, and it can just as easily learn a new association.

You might react to triggers for a while, but with practice, those reactions might only last for milliseconds.

Tool 4.1: Identify triggers

Date:

To identify your triggers, consider each sense: sight, hearing, smell, taste, and touch. You might be surprised at how many there are. Be honest and list them all—even if they seem insignificant. If there's more than one behavior you want to change, list them all in the left column.

Behavior	**Triggers**
Ex: Gambling	Lottery ads; scratch-off tickets in stores
Ex: Drinking alcohol	Attending a wedding; Being offered a free beer at the end of a 5k run

Tool 4.2: Rank trigger risks

Date:

Not all triggers are equally powerful. Some are uniquely more likely to create an urge for you than others. Rate each trigger from 1 (weakest) to 10 (riskiest). Then, you can prioritize the triggers you most need to be prepared for. Key categories are listed below. Add your own from Tool 4.1.

Trigger	**Rating (1-10)**
Unpleasant emotions (ex: anger, frustration, grief) Others:	
Pleasant emotions (ex: joy, peace, anticipation) Others:	
Physical sensations (ex: pain, cold, heat) Others:	
Stress (ex: deadlines, anxiety, financial concerns) Others:	
Conflicts with others (ex: coworker, partner, family) Others:	
Places and times (ex: restaurants, cars, summer, weekends) Others:	
Other:	
Other:	
Other:	
Other:	

Tool 4.3: Log your urges

Date:

Do you know how long your urges last? Or when they're strongest? By writing them down, you'll begin to see patterns.
If you keep a journal, you can keep it with you and record your urges there. At first, you might jot down many urges per day—that's normal.

Date	Time	Strength (1-10)	Length of Urge	What triggered my urge?	Who/where was involved?	How I coped and felt about it	Ideas for next time
8/29	1:15 pm	8	1 minute	Lunch in a wine bar	Lisa and Stephanie	Told them and forgot pretty fast	Find a new lunch spot

Reflecting on your urges, what hidden triggers do you identify? Do any recurring thought patterns emerge? What places, people, or activities can you avoid or distract yourself from?

More copies on page 89

Dealing with discomfort

Now you probably understand your urges better. You know what activates them, when they typically arise, and how strong they are. The next question is: How do you deal with them and the discomfort they bring?

Discomfort can be physical, emotional, or both. What we believe about discomfort affects how much it influences us. If you don't think you should have to deal with discomfort, it can make it harder to bear. But discomfort is a normal part of life. You've built powerful, habitual responses to discomfort. It's instinctive, like shifting your weight from one foot to another while you're waiting in line.

Some situations aren't what you want them to be. But discomfort isn't always bad. It can be a useful feeling. Discomfort can tell us something is wrong and motivate us to change the situation (or our thinking about it).

Types of discomfort

- **Physical pain.** Believing that pain shouldn't exist only adds to the discomfort.
- **Withdrawal.** When you're in withdrawal, despair or depression can creep in. It won't last forever, and addictive behavior isn't the only solution.
- **Preoccupation/Anticipation.** Even if you're not in withdrawal, you may begin thinking ahead to engaging in your addictive behavior again.
- **Anxiety.** Anxiety kept our ancestors vigilant against the dangers of a wilder and more uncertain world. It's stronger in some people than others, but it's natural. Believing the world must be made safe adds to discomfort.
- **Depression.** Biology and heredity can be a major contributor to depression that requires medical treatment. But for many, depression comes from the demands we place on ourselves, others, and the world. For example, if you believe you must be universally loved or successful to be happy, you'll find yourself unhappy a lot.
- **Frustration and anger.** These can come from a mismatch in how you want yourself to perform and how you do perform. They can also come from how you think others should behave versus how they do.

Learn to recognize these feelings for what they are: types of discomfort. They're sensations that will pass, not a reason to return to your old patterns of behavior.

Strategies for coping with urges

How exactly you deal with the discomfort of an urge can vary from person to person. Some strategies may work better for you than others. Try the ones you gravitate to and keep note of what works best.

Basic strategies[2]

- **Avoid.** Stay away from triggers that lead to urges.
- **Escape.** If you find yourself in a triggering situation, leave right away.
- **Distract yourself.** Concentrate on something you enjoy. See the list on page 42 for ideas.
- **Talk yourself through it.** If something upsets you, you might think you deserve a break from your new pattern of behavior. Instead, try telling yourself it sucks, but that a break isn't going to fix the situation.
- **Revisit your motivation.** Think about the future you imagined or the cost-benefit analysis you did in Point 1. You might still be uncomfortable, and that'll keep you committed.
- **Rate your urge.** Put the moment in perspective and ask yourself whether you're exaggerating. Compare the discomfort to something tangible, like having your hair pulled or stepping on a piece of glass. You might even make yourself laugh.
- **Recall a moment of clarity.** Think back to a time when your commitment to stop was crystal-clear. Where were you? What were your thoughts?
- **Remember the cons.** Imagine you give in to your urge. Follow it through: What consequences follow? Say you want a cigarette. Remind yourself about coughing as you use the stairs and not only the smoke itself.
- **Picture your future.** Visualize yourself in the near future, feeling good about resisting. What will tomorrow be like?
- **Use past successes.** Remember a time you successfully resisted an urge. Find confidence in that and remind yourself the urge will pass.
- **Ride the wave.** Imagine yourself surfing a wave that grows, crests, weakens, and disappears from view.
- **Talk to others.** Talk to someone who's overcome urges and get tips. SMART meetings are filled with people who can encourage and support you.
- **Get social support.** Talk with a nonjudgmental and supportive person you know. You might want to keep a list of these people handy. Let them know how they can help you, since they might not realize their role.
- **Accept and acknowledge the urge.** Accept the urge as uncomfortable and experience it as a passing thought. Acknowledge it as something that used to be a problem, then get back to what you were doing.
- **Role play.** Urges often arise in social situations. It can be helpful to prepare for those situations. "Role play" is one way to prepare. In role play you and others play out the roles of a social situation. You could role play in a SMART meeting, with a friend, or by yourself (you play all the roles).

[2] From Sex, Drugs, Gambling & Chocolate: A Workbook for Overcoming Addictions by Thomas Horvath

In the role play you go back and forth, you and one or more people. Here's an example:

Friend: Would you like to have dessert?

Me: No thanks

Friend: That's funny, you usually have dessert.

Me: True, but not tonight.

Friend: Why not? Does that mean I have to eat dessert alone?

Me: You can order dessert if you want to. I'm just not going to have any.

Friend: OK, maybe I should do the same.

In this example your friend pushes back only a little. You can practice many rounds of role play, each one getting a little harder.

The role play exercise can be a very stimulating and fun exercise in a SMART meeting.

Distraction ideas

What distractions are healthy for you will depend on the behavior you're working to change. Highlight or circle ones that might help you and add your own. Some of these may become passions in time!

Category	Examples
Learn something new	Learn art, history, languages, math, science, humanities
Arts	Draw, write, paint, take photos, sculpt
Books and entertainment	Read, listen to live music, go to a movie or live show, watch TV
Chores	Clean, cook, wash dishes, iron, garden, do laundry
Crafts	Knit, embroider, scrapbook, do woodworking
Exercise	Walk, run, swim, do yoga, ski, do martial arts, lift weights, go skating
Games	Play board games, cards, darts, puzzles, mental challenges (ex: say the alphabet backwards)
Outdoor activities	Watch birds, hike, walk, bike
Performing arts and music	Sing, practice an instrument, mime, dance
Personal growth	Read, attend a meeting, learn a new skill, go to a lecture
Religion and spirituality	Attend a service, pray, meditate, attend a study group
Socializing	Attend a meet-up, go to a group or club, make plans with a friend
Sports	Play or watch table tennis, hockey, soccer, softball, kickball
Trades and crafts	Paint, work on a car, tinker
Vent feelings	Talk, journal, cry, throw eggs at the ground
Volunteer	Soup kitchen, hospice, church, SMART

Tool 4.4: Plan your week

Sometimes having a plan for your week can help you avoid triggering situations. Try adding healthy distractions and activities throughout your week.

Time	Monday	Tuesday	Wednesday	Thursday	Friday	Saturday	Sunday
Morning							
Midday							
Evening							

Memory trick: Put DENTS in your urges

DENTS is an easy way to remember strategies for managing urges. And that's important, because urges can make it hard to think clearly.

Deny or delay	Remind yourself as many times as you need to that this urge will pass. Refuse to give in, no matter what—even if that means delaying by one moment at a time.
Escape	If you know what is triggering your urge, leave immediately or end the trigger.
Neutralize	You can neutralize an urge in a few ways. You can attack it and prove it wrong (see Tool 5.1 in the next chapter). Or you can acknowledge it and let it pass. Create emotional distance by watching the urge build, crest, and fade. Don't pretend it doesn't exist, just recognize that it exists and is separate from you.
Tasks	Give yourself something to do. When you put your mind on something else, it can't focus on the urge. Try the distractions on page 42 or a simple activity like counting or reciting.
Swap	Change your internal monologue or thinking. Instead of "This urge will kill me," think "This urge will pass." If you feel sad or lonely, deliberately change it by going to the gym or having a laugh.

Tool 4.5: Customize DENTS for you

DENTS (page 46) can help you remember how to get through an urge. Once you're familiar with it, write down what strategies help you in each row.

Deny or delay	How long do urges last if you don't give in? How bad do they get before they fade?
Escape	What triggers can you get away from? How can you minimize their influence?
Neutralize	What techniques help you sit with urges until they pass? What words or SMART activities provide comfort?
Tasks	What activities absorb you fully enough to fend off urges?
Swap	What positive thoughts chase out your negative ones during an urge? What healthy activities clear your mind?

Tool 4.6: Personify and disarm

Date:	
The urges you feel aren't you. They're an impulse or a reaction—something separate from you. For some, personifying urges can create a helpful boundary. It also helps something abstract feel more concrete and manageable.	
Name	Ex: The whiner, the lobbyist, the hurt child
What you say or do to them	Ex: I see you and I am in control here; I hear you and don't need your help anymore.
What happens when you say it	Ex: They lose their power, they dissolve, they move on

Tip: Rejecting pressure

If someone pressures you to engage in your addictive behavior, try these tips:

- Make eye contact. It shows you're serious.
- Speak in a firm, unhesitating voice.
- Don't feel guilty. You have the right to choose.
- After you say no, change the subject. Don't entertain continued pressure.

Advanced strategies

The basic strategies above are designed to help you in the moment. When you feel more confident, you might try these advanced strategies. These are meant to enhance your ability to resist urges when you have some time to prepare.

Strategy	What to do	How to cope
Move past avoidance Avoidance is a great early strategy but not always realistic long term. This strategy helps you build the confidence to resist direct invitations to old behaviors.	Put yourself in a situation that may trigger an urge, like going to a bar or club. It may help to bring along a trusted companion for support and guidance.	Use any basic strategies you like. Practice refusing offers and peer pressure. Visualize someone trying to persuade you or making fun of you for saying no. Maybe it's someone who usually knows how to get to you. Then, visualize yourself confidently refusing and staying focused.
Bring out an urge Confront an urge on your terms instead of waiting for one to arise. This strategy works best when you already have some mastery over urges.	Remember a strong urge you had in the past. (Maybe check your urge log.) You can also imagine a situation you expect to happen in the future.	Visualize yourself giving into the urge, and let it pass. Then visualize the same situation, but resist the urge. Do this for as many situations as you find helpful.
Prepare for social situations If you expect an upcoming event to trigger you—like a party or get-together—use this strategy to minimize its impact.	Talk with another person about the event beforehand. Update them afterward. If you trust the host, enlist them as an ally. Before you go, tell them what you're avoiding, so they can help.	Arrive late and leave early. Prepare an escape plan, including reasons to leave. Get something to hold—like a club soda—right away. Others will be less inclined to offer you something. Remember that nobody's paying as much attention to you as you imagine.
Analyze the activating event, your beliefs, and the consequences	We'll cover this technique in Point 3: Managing feelings, thoughts, and behaviors.	

Chapter Summary

- Urges are a part of the journey to reduce addictive behaviors for most people.
- Acting on an urge is a choice. We act on urges to gain immediate satisfaction or alleviate discomfort.
- Discomfort is subjective and normal. Thinking we shouldn't have to deal with discomfort can make us more uncomfortable.
- If we give up some immediate satisfaction, we may be able to increase other types of satisfaction in our lives.
- Although urges can come up quickly, the tools to respond to them may require planning and practice.

Chapter 5
Point 3: Managing thoughts, feelings, and behaviors

Like addictive behaviors, thinking can become automatic. Some habitual thoughts are uncomfortable ones. They can make addictive behaviors seem like comforting retreats.

In this chapter, we'll guide you through tools that can help you respond differently to your thinking. When you can do that, your emotions and behaviors will likely also change.

Downing beliefs

Downing beliefs are negative thoughts about ourselves, others, or our lives. They make us feel guilty, ashamed, depressed, or angry. An example would be saying to yourself, "I messed up again. I'm a total failure." Downing beliefs are an exaggeration. As humans, we're prone to making them. And they can upset us in ways that trap us in a cycle of addictive behavior.

Practicing unconditional acceptance – for yourself, others, and life in general – is a way to challenge downing beliefs and reduce their impact.

Unconditional acceptance

Unconditional acceptance is the belief that something has worth just as it is. Adopting this belief is a life skill that can help you far beyond the context of your current change process.

Unconditional acceptance is easier to preach than practice. To adopt it, practice recognizing unhelpful beliefs when they arise. That's typically when something unpleasant or unexpected happens in your life. Once you spot those beliefs, you can remind yourself of more helpful beliefs.

Unconditional self-acceptance

Unconditional self-acceptance is recognizing that you have worth just as you are. When you do this, you separate yourself from your behaviors. You are a collection of your character, traits, personality, strengths, and weaknesses. You are not your behaviors and your behaviors can change. You'll still be you.

This is why SMART doesn't encourage the use of labels. You may engage in an addictive behavior, but "addict" doesn't summarize you. It might seem like a game of words, but words and labels are powerful. You might have attached other negative labels to yourself, like "failure," "disappointment," or "weak." If you don't accept yourself, others won't either. Or, if they do accept you, can you believe them, believing what you do about yourself?

To help build unconditional self-acceptance:

- **Remind yourself you're human.** Humans aren't perfect. We make mistakes, do some things badly, and do some bad things. Making mistakes and failing is how we learn.
- **Replace negative thoughts.** Correct exaggerations you make about yourself. When you do, you'll feel better and want to act in healthier ways.
- **Be patient and kind with yourself.** Accept that you can't change the past, but you can create your future. Even if you caused pain to yourself or others, you can forgive yourself, even if others won't.
- **Don't compare yourself to others or an arbitrary standard.** There is no standard measure of your value. You're the only you. Comparing yourself to others is like judging one color against another. Is red good or bad? Is blue more valuable than green?

After practicing this for a while, more accurate thinking will become automatic for you. Like most things, though, it takes practice.

Unconditional acceptance of others

We can judge others in exaggerated ways too. You're capable of making mistakes, and others are too. Judging someone else as totally bad is an exaggeration. It can be just as damaging as judging yourself, because it's not the whole truth.

It can be especially difficult to accept someone who treats you badly. You can accept that they're human, even if you don't accept their behavior. Sometimes that means acknowledging that we can't change or control them. With that acceptance, you may choose to practice communicating healthy boundaries or remove yourself from a relationship.

Unconditional life acceptance

We can also misjudge our lives as completely unfair or totally terrible. We all occasionally find ourselves thinking, "Life sucks! It couldn't be more awful!" Remind yourself that good things have happened in your life too.

Try to accept that there are many things in life you can't control. This can help you to keep those in perspective, even if you don't like something that happened.

Helpful and unhelpful beliefs

Beliefs may be categorized as helpful, unhelpful, or somewhere in between. You can explore how helpful or unhelpful a belief is.

Helpful beliefs
are true, make sense, or are helpful.

Unhelpful beliefs
aren't true, don't make sense, or are unhelpful

Types of unhelpful beliefs

These types of unhelpful beliefs are associated with uncomfortable feelings that may fuel addictive behaviors. Do you recognize any?

Belief type	**What to listen for**	**The problem**
Demands	Must Have to	"I have to make this work." These put rigid and unrealistic demands on you, others, or your life. They create emotional distress when they're not met, or even when you doubt they will be.
Overgeneralizations	Only Always Never	"Things never go the way I want." "I only get heartbreak." "My partner always complains that I'm not here enough." These are all-or-nothing ways of thinking. Reality usually falls somewhere in between. Life is filled with gray areas and unknowns, even if you wish it wasn't.
Frustration intolerance	Can't	"I can't deal with this anymore." There's a lot you do deal with, handle, or put up with. You may not always do it in a healthy way, but you're still here.
Awfulizations	Worst Most Words that end in "-est," (like stupidest or cruelest)	"This is the worst thing that's ever happened to me." "This is the most frustrating thing in the world." How many times have you applied this belief to an unpleasant situation? How often has it been true?

Unhelpful beliefs can all become reasons to engage in our addictive behavior.
Take time to examine your thinking. Ask yourself:

- What evidence do I have to support this belief?
- How true is it?
- What's a more balanced way of looking at this?

Common unhelpful beliefs

Feel free to highlight or circle any beliefs that tend to lead you to engage with your addictive behavior.

Unhelpful belief	Question	Helpful belief
I always fail.	Have I never succeeded at anything?	I've done some things well in the past, so I don't and won't always fail.
I'm totally worthless.	Have I never done anything worthwhile?	I have done some dumb things. But I've succeeded at some worthwhile things. So, no, I'm not totally worthless.
My partner treats me unfairly and is a bad person.	Has my partner ever done something helpful for me?	My partner has been unfair, but they've also helped me. Nobody is perfect, so I won't judge them as a totally bad person.
Nothing good ever happens to me and never will.	Can I think of a time where something good did happen for me?	The love and support of my family and friends are all good things that continue to happen to me.
I must be comfortable at all times.	Is it realistic to expect to always feel comfortable?	Comfort ebbs and flows. It may be better to stay uncomfortable temporarily if it will help me achieve my long-term goals.
Messing up proves I'm a complete failure.	Am I the only human being who makes mistakes?	I don't judge others as harshly as I judge myself. Everyone makes mistakes. I can make mistakes and learn from them. That makes me human, not a failure.
I have to be better and do better than the people around me or I am nothing.	Am I only what I do and how well I do it?	I don't need to prove I'm better than others to be OK. I can be happy just as I am. I deserve to accept myself.

Unhelpful belief	Question	Helpful belief
My addictive behavior proves I should never trust myself or my instincts. I will always need the advice of others.	What are some good choices I've made for myself?	I've made mistakes and will continue to make them. But I can learn which thoughts and feelings to trust. I don't need others' opinions to validate my self-worth, even while I might benefit from input about the decisions I make.
Others are responsible for my unhappiness. I hate them, I want to punish them, or I deserve to complain bitterly when they disappoint me.	Are other people in charge of my happiness?	I'm responsible for my happiness. Holding others responsible is unrealistic and unfair. It doesn't lead to my long-term happiness.
I must find the one person or belief that will make my life stable.	Is there one person or belief that will make me happy?	Life is an ongoing process of learning and relating to many people. It's a journey on which I will change and grow. What helps me now can change.
I'm bored, and that makes me uncomfortable. The only thing I can do is engage in my addictive behavior.	Is engaging in my addictive behavior the only option I have?	I can do other things to relieve boredom. It'll get my mind off the addictive behavior.

Tool 5.1: Dispute unhelpful beliefs

Date:

Refer to the table of common unhelpful beliefs (page 52) or write down your own. Then, question the belief and provide a more reasonable alternative.

My unhelpful belief	Question	Helpful belief
Ex: I can't deal with this without using.	Can I deal with it?	It might be hard, but I can. It's going to get easier.

More copies on page 89

Changing your vocabulary

We can't control what thoughts, emotions or situations arise in our lives. But we can describe them in ways that don't add to our discomfort. You might be surprised by how much the words matter. Try the substitutions below for a while. See which ones become natural.

Instead of:	Try this:
Words	
Must, should, ought to	Really want Prefer Choose to
Have to	Want to
Can't	Choose not to
Awful	Not great Not what I want
Unbearable	Unpleasant
Can't stand	Don't like
Always	Often
All	A lot
Statements	
I must be perfect	I really want to do well
You shouldn't do that	I prefer you not do that
You should help	I'd appreciate your help
I can't stand this feeling	I don't like feeling this way
You're a bad person	I don't like what you're doing
This urge is awful	This urge is uncomfortable
This situation is unbearable	This isn't the best way
Everything is terrible	Things aren't the way I want them to be
This happens every time	This happens a lot

I need your love	I want to be loved
I'm a bad person	I regret how I acted
I'm a failure	I made a mistake I didn't succeed this time
Emotions	
I'm anxious	I feel concerned
I'm depressed	I feel sad
I'm angry	I feel annoyed
I'm guilty I'm ashamed	I feel regret I feel disappointment
I'm jealous I'm envious	I feel concern about my relationship I feel unhappy

Managing feelings

Strong emotions are inevitable. Whether they're considered "good" or "bad," strong emotions can result in us behaving in self-defeating ways.

Let's use anger as an example. Low-level annoyance can lead to positive and assertive action. It might help you stand up for yourself or others in the face of injustice. Unbridled rage, on the other hand, can be dangerous and destructive. Annoyance provides an opportunity for balance and reflection, while rage reduces our ability to think clearly.

Learning to reduce extreme emotions by adjusting your beliefs could make it easier to change how you act.

Changing your beliefs

Rational emotive behavior therapy outlines the ABCs of a given event. We can use the ABCs to reduce that event's power over us.[3] Mapping the ABCs can help you work through uncomfortable thoughts and feelings, including urges. It's a tool that can help you think and feel better in all aspects of your life—not just in your current change process.

[3] Ellis, Albert (1975). A Guide to Rational Living. Wilshire Book Company.

What are the ABCs?

Activating event	Something happens in your life. It could be a behavior of someone else, or even a thought or an emotion that arises within yourself. Let's say, for example, that your boss yells at you.
Beliefs about the event	• What you believe about A. The beliefs could be helpful, unhelpful, or a mixture of both. In the example of a boss yelling at you, beliefs that could arise include: • I am a failure. • I can't stand someone being upset with me. • This isn't fair. • Engaging in my addictive behavior is the only way I can deal with the shame I'm feeling.
Consequences of your beliefs	• What you feel or how you behave in response to A because of B. In the example of a boss yelling at you, you might: • Quit your job • Angrily tell everyone you know what a monster your boss is • Engage in your addictive behavior

Putting the ABCs into practice

When you're first learning the ABCs, it can help to start with C (the consequence). Typically, the consequence is the easiest thing to identify, and it might include engaging in your addictive behavior. The A (the activating event) might also come easily—what triggered you? What made you feel an intense emotion that you wanted relief from? Now you can analyze B (beliefs). What beliefs got you automatically from A to C?

Adding D and E

It's B (your beliefs) that actually lead to C (consequences), not A. Maybe you can't change A (the activating event). No matter: You can control your beliefs about it. By changing your beliefs, you change how you feel about it, and that changes how you react. Now that you know the ABCs of a situation, you can move on to D and E.

Dispute your beliefs	Ask yourself how true the beliefs you identified are. What demands are unrealistic? Where are you refusing to tolerate frustration? Look for evidence to support each belief. (Discomfort alone doesn't make them true.)
Effective new belief	Now, replace the unhelpful beliefs with more helpful ones. For example: • I really want to use when I feel like this. And I don't have to. • This is unpleasant, and I can sit with the discomfort until it passes. My urge won't kill me, and it isn't unbearable.

When you understand that these new and effective beliefs are true, your discomfort may subside or decrease, reducing the urge's intensity. You may identify beliefs that seem very difficult to change. You could bring them up in a meeting. The group will not tell you what to believe. However, you may hear helpful beliefs from others that you had not thought of.

Do you remember the quote from Epictetus earlier in this handbook? "We are disturbed not by events but by our views about them." One of the fundamental aspects of SMART is realizing that we can view ourselves, our situations, and our futures differently. The ABC tool is one way to put that realization into practice.

Tool 5.2: ABC exercise

Date:

Activating event	**B**elief about the event	**C**onsequence of the unhelpful belief	**D**ispute the unhelpful belief	**E**ffective thinking change
The event that created the urge.	What I unhelpfully believe about A—the "must."	How I feel and behave in response to A because of B.	Questions I ask myself to dispute the unhelpful belief B	The new more effective belief I adopt to replace B, which leads to a different C in response to A.
Ex: My boss yelled at me today in front of my coworkers.	He has no right to embarrass me. It's not fair. I can't stand this.	I'm really mad and I want a drink.	Does my boss only yell at me? Is life always fair? Can I stand this without a drink?	My boss yells at everyone sooner or later. Life isn't fair. That didn't feel great, and it's over. My boss isn't worth giving up my long-term goals.

More copies on page 89

Coping during a crisis

In moments of crisis, you won't have time to work through the ABCs. They take time and some detachment from the situation. Coping statements are another strategy. These are statements (or mantras) you say to yourself to get through the moment. You can do an ABC later.

It's helpful to develop and rehearse a few coping statements so they're ready when you need them. Make your coping statements realistic ones that don't put demands on yourself or others.

The table of common unhelpful beliefs (page 54-55) can provide a starting point.
Here are a few others that align with common uncomfortable emotions:

For frustration

- I'm frustrated. I don't like this, and it won't kill me. I can handle what I don't like without saying something I'll regret.
- This is upsetting, and I can stand what I don't like.

For anger or rage:

- I'm really angry. It's OK to feel this way and I don't have to act on my feelings.
- I don't have to lash out when someone acts badly toward me. It's OK to feel annoyed.

For anxiety, depression, or grief:

- I can't change what happened, and I can learn how to respond differently.
- I made a mistake. I'm human. I'm forgiving myself and moving on.

You can find more coping statements with a simple web search.

Problem solving

We work on our beliefs and get better at managing our thoughts, feelings, and behaviors.
Still, we may find that some external problems in our life remain.

Addictive behaviors may seem like a solution to some problems. When those other problems are overwhelming, avoiding them is especially appealing. But addictive behaviors don't solve those other problems at all: They mask them. Learning problem-solving strategies can help you approach the problems themselves confidently.

Managing problems becomes easier if you can accept that:

- Some people will not accept that you have changed.
- Some situations will be beyond your control.

These aren't problems you can solve. They're facts of life. For other problems you encounter, you can start by working in small, manageable steps.

Five-step problem solving

1. Define the problem	Be careful not to assume a symptom is the root of the problem. One common technique is "asking the 5 whys"—asking "why" 5 times, or until you reach the root of the problem. Your problem may be straightforward: You've been evicted; therefore, you need a new place to live. Others may be harder: Your daughter keeps running away.
2. Brainstorm solutions	Come up with as many ideas as you can. They don't all need to be good. Some may even be bizarre or wild. Just let them flow. You can do this alone, with a friend or therapist, or in a SMART meeting. The important part is that you don't judge the ideas prematurely. Stop yourself from saying "That won't work," or "I've tried that before, and..."
3. Evaluate the options	Rate each idea from 0 (unlikely to work) to 10 (a fantastic option). Consider these criteria: • Is this realistic? • Is it likely to work? • Does it have rewards? • What are its consequences? • Can I afford it? Check your assumptions before you jump to a conclusion.
4. Pick one	You've thought the problem through. Choose one and try it. You can always go back and try a different option if the first one doesn't work out.
5. Create a plan	It's tempting to carry the solution around in your head. But if you write it down, you may get better results. Break your solution into steps. What do you need to do first? And next? You might want to write down important locations, dates, or supplies. Use the change-plan worksheet (Tool 3.4 on page 31) if it helps.

Tool 5.3: Practice problem solving

Date:	
Use this Tool to explore how you might solve a large or small problem. Refer to the five-step problem-solving guide on page 65.	
What is the root of the problem?	
How could I address the problem?	
Idea: 1. 2. 3. 4. 5.	**Likeliness to work (0-10):** 1. 2. 3. 4. 5.
Which idea will I try?	
What individual steps should I take as part of my plan? You can also refer to Tool 3.4, the change-plan worksheet, on page 31.	
More copies on page 89	

Putting your choice into action

Problem solving requires the three Ps:

- **Practice**
- **Patience**
- **Persistence**

You have a choice. You're ready to try it. Now you observe how it's working.

Record your results every day if helpful. Your results might be different from what you wanted or expected. How can you adjust? Should you try a different option? You can ask for thoughts or feedback from a SMART meeting or friend as you go.

Like most things, this takes practice. Eventually your intuition and confidence will build. Find people who will give you honest feedback while supporting you. You'll make mistakes, and that's OK. Try not to get discouraged. Remember that though a particular solution may fail, that doesn't make you a failure.

Healthy Communication in Relationships

Supportive and healthy relationships can be an asset in your process of change. Communicating positively with others and setting healthy boundaries for yourself can help you build, or rebuild, healthy relationships. The more effectively you're able to communicate with family, friends, and other loved ones, the more likely their support of you will feel helpful.

Many find it hard to communicate with their loved ones in a way that benefits and nurtures both parties. Communication erodes more quickly when relationships are troubled. And where addictive behaviors are involved, that's often the case.

In a troubled situation, both people start to make negative comments instead of positive ones. "You statements" start replacing "I-statements." Each person starts to disregard the other's point of view. Eventually, each blames the other.

Here are two tools from the SMART Family & Friends program that may help you communicate more effectively—with your loved ones, but also everyone else, too!

Tool 5.4: Planning positive conversations

<table>
<tr><td colspan="2">When planning for a potentially challenging conversation with someone you care about, consider PIVA.</td></tr>
<tr><td>P</td><td>Positive framing of your request increases the chance that you'll be heard.

It helps you both remember what you appreciate about the other person. Tell them something you like about them. Or just tell them you love them. Tell them what you want, not what you don't want.</td></tr>
<tr><td>I</td><td>I-statements reduce the chance of defensiveness getting in the way.

I-statements communicate our needs and wishes without blaming or criticizing the other person. For example, instead of saying "You make me so sad," you can say "I feel sad when you yell at me."

When you're making a request, you can use I-statements too: "I'd like to ask you to tell me how you're feel without yelling at me."</td></tr>
<tr><td>V</td><td>Validate what you can.

Show your loved one you care about them and respect them by trying to understand their point of view, even if you don't agree with it. Validate what you can—especially their feelings. Really listen. Ask questions and clarify what you think you've heard.</td></tr>
<tr><td>A</td><td>Ask how you can help.

Neither one of you is perfect. Understanding and acknowledging your role in a problematic pattern of behavior can help diffuse conflicts.</td></tr>
</table>

Healthy boundaries

In healthy relationships, boundaries are negotiated smoothly in the background. They form the basis for mutual respect between two people, and you may never think about them. You may never say them out loud.

Healthy boundaries aren't about the other person or their actions. They are about ourselves. They're ways we stay true to our values and direction. They remind us (and others) that we have value. Our trust, affection, time, energy, health, and friendship have value, and we'll protect those things. Healthy boundaries are a sign of respect for ourselves and our desires.

Unhealthy boundaries

When a relationship becomes unhealthy, boundaries are often a central issue. Others can push us to give up or suppress our own values. We sometimes let our boundaries slide to keep the peace or maintain a relationship.

What boundaries are and aren't

Boundaries aren't brick walls—they're fences. They mark out personal space, rights, and preferences. They're not a way to keep people out. It's not feasible to have a relationship with someone on the other side of a solid brick wall. But it's very possible to have a relationship with someone on the other side of a gated fence

Communicating a boundary effectively

Communicating directly and honestly is critical. It's how we demonstrate respect for ourselves and others. Since our boundaries are about us and not others, it's best to make them I-statements. This format tends to work well:

I feel __________ when you __________.	**Can I ask you to ______________?**
Inform	Request

Examples

- "I feel frustrated when you have the TV turned up loud because I can't hear the baby monitor. Can I ask you to please turn the volume down?"
- "I feel embarrassed when you confront me about my drinking in front of others. Can I ask that we have those conversations in private?"

While wording the request as a question acknowledges that the other person has a choice, some people prefer to word the request as a statement. For example, "I need you to turn the TV down please" or "Please call and let me know you will be late" in the examples above.

Similarly, you may find that rewording the Inform statement to eliminate the word "you" is helpful. In the examples above, this might look like "I feel frustrated with the TV loud because I can't hear the baby monitor" and "I feel worried when I don't know where you are."

There is no right or wrong way to word your boundary requests. You get to decide the language that works for you and your loved one.

Tool 5.5: Setting healthy boundaries

You can build confidence by communicating small boundaries before you broach big ones. What small boundaries can you begin setting? It's a good idea to practice on people in your life who aren't closest to you, too.

What small boundaries would you like to communicate?

Who	What	How
Ex: Colleague	Wash own coffee mugs	I feel frustrated when you don't wash your own coffee mug. Can I ask you to please start doing that?

What larger boundaries might you want to communicate with some practice?

Who	What	How

Staying on track

A lapse is a short slip into an old behavior. It's an isolated incident. You could experience a prolonged return to your old pattern of addictive behavior, sometimes called a "relapse." Some people prefer to refer to both lapses and relapses by the more neutral phrases "return to an old pattern of behavior" or "returns to use." As stated previously, you get to choose the language that's helpful for you.

Returns to an old pattern of behavior can happen at any time. They can even happen once you consider your addictive behavior resolved. They are more likely to happen in high stress situations in your life. Some tips for these situations:

- Think carefully and honestly about how vulnerable you are. Stay vigilant.
- Remember where you've been and what you've achieved.
- Consider doing an ABC worksheet (Tool 5.2, page 61) on "I've regained complete control and don't need to be cautious anymore."
- Go to a meeting and discuss what occurred, even if you haven't been to a meeting in a while.

Whatever language you use to think about your addictive behavior patterns, well-established patterns have staying power. Once they return, they don't want to go away.

However long a lapse or relapse lasts, it can still be temporary. You can learn from the experience and recall the progress that you've made so far. Consider talking about what happened in your next meeting and develop more strategies to avoid another lapse.

Additional high-risk situations

Lapses and relapses can happen without you feeling an urge. Prevention is the best way to avoid them. Watch out for these five high risk situations and any others that are relevant for you:

- **Association.** You're exposed to a past trigger.
- **Boredom.** This kind of discomfort can let old thinking patterns return.
- **Strong emotions.** An unexpected wave of frustration, anger, or grief can send you back to old ways of coping.
- **Fantasy.** Once you have some distance, you might romanticize the fun parts of an addictive behavior.
- **Opportunity.** This is a moment when it seems like there's no downside to engaging in the behavior. Maybe no one else will know, but you will.

When you see one of these coming up, consider rehearsing how you'll react. (See the advanced strategies on page 49 for some ideas.)

Tools for staying on track

Practice any of the techniques in Point 2: Coping with urges, including distraction, DENTS, and others. These will help you think about any cravings realistically. Although staying on track can be challenging at first, it often gets easier with regular practice.

- **Treat underlying illness.** If you need medical or psychological help, get it. Untreated problems can make addictive behaviors appealing. Take medications as prescribed.
- **Stay wary of excessive immediate satisfaction.** Build up the habit of not acting on urges without thinking about them. Regularly review and update motivations you developed in Point 1: Finding and maintaining motivation. This includes your values, five questions, and cost-benefit analysis. Remember: You are building up the habit of living your life according to your values.
- **Reward yourself.** Choose a reward that furthers one of your healthy passions, like one related to the distractions on page 46.

Whatever tools you choose to use to stay on track, know that you are welcome to discuss your journey in our meetings. Additional tools may be made available on the SMART Recovery website from time to time.

Chapter Summary

- Unhelpful beliefs can result in unhelpful automatic thoughts, feelings, and behaviors, including addictive behaviors.
- Learning to adopt more helpful beliefs can reduce uncomfortable emotions and unhelpful behaviors. Then you can respond more effectively to all types of challenging things that may happen in your life.
- Techniques like the ABC tool (Tool 5.2, page 61) and disputing unhelpful beliefs (Tool 5.1, page 56) can help you behave in more effective ways going forward.

Chapter 6
Point 4: Living a balanced life

In chapter 2, we explained that the process of change is not only about reducing or resolving an addictive behavior. It's about your wellness, empowerment, and potential. It involves regaining your health and creating a lifestyle that brings you satisfaction. This comes from finding and pursuing interests that absorb you. It also comes from setting and achieving long-term goals.

Many people live out of balance, in ways that are at odds with their values. (Now's a good time to revisit yours from page 29). Achieving balance takes work.

Two things can help create balance:

- Understanding and respecting each area of your life
- Changing your perspective in the areas where you feel stuck

See Tool 6.1 on the following page.

Tool 6.1: Check your lifestyle balance (lifestyle balance wheel[4])

Date:

Each spoke of the wheel represents an area of your life. Examples include family, friends, spirituality, romance, health, career, and finances. Some of your values (page 29) might also appear.

Rate your satisfaction (not how much energy you spend) in each aspect of your life by putting a dot on the center line. The outside edge is totally satisfied, while the inner corner is totally unsatisfied. Then connect the dots and see what shape you get. The rounder the wheel, the more balanced your life is.

See an example and tips on the next pages.

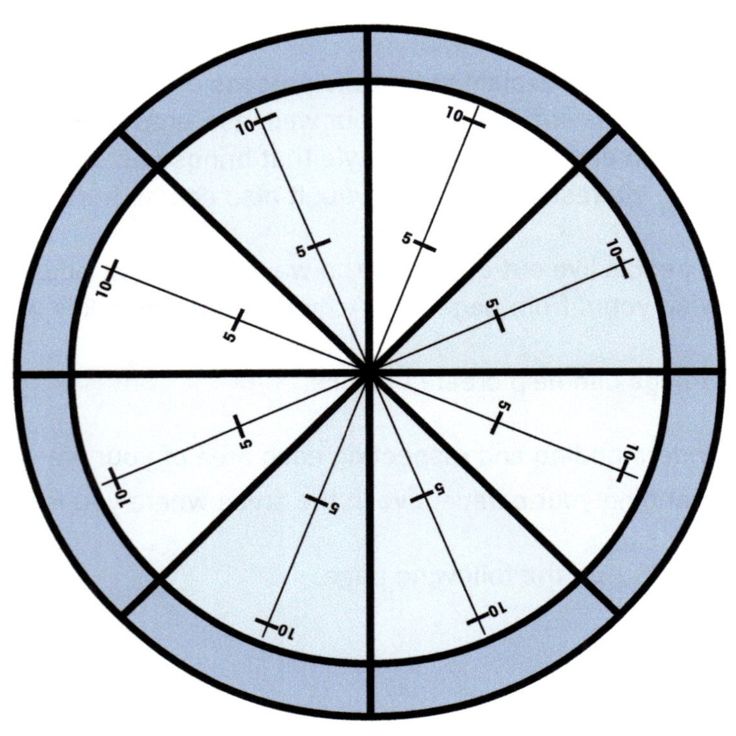

Highest-scoring categories	Lowest-scoring categories
1	8
2	7
3	6
4	5
Ask yourself: • Would this wheel roll? • What areas need more or less attention? • How well does my wheel reflect my values? • Am I involved in too much? • How much time do I spend caring for others? For myself?	**Notes and plans:**

More copies on page 89

[4] This exercise and graphic are based on the work of Julia Cameron's The Artist's Way. Used by permission from Penguin Publishers.

EXAMPLE

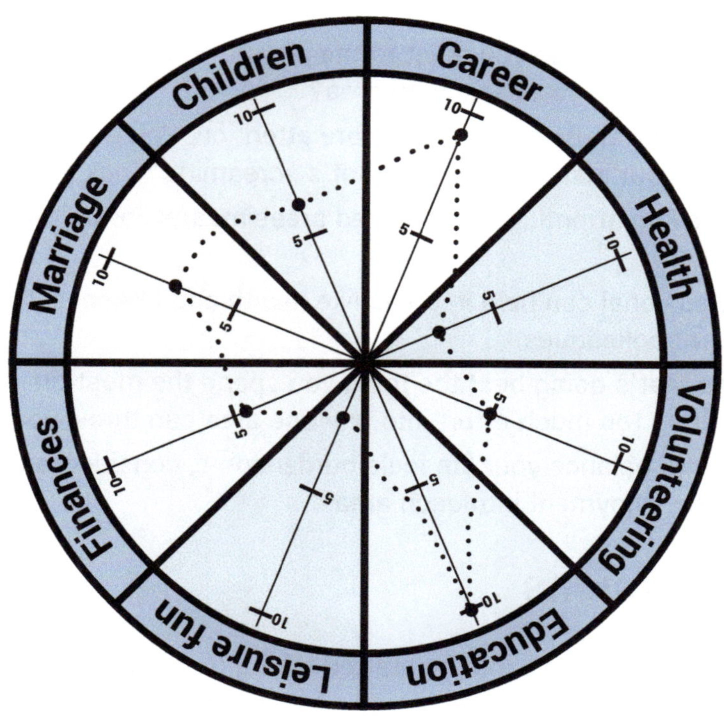

Highest-scoring categories	Lowest-scoring categories
1. Children	8. Leisure/fun
2. Marriage	7. Health
3. Career	6. Finances
4. Education	5. Volunteering

Notes and plans:

My leisure/fun and health areas scored lowest. To increase both, I'll join a walking club. When I seem confident in these areas, I'll move on to finances and volunteering.

Changing your lifestyle balance

Reflect on your lifestyle balance in these ways:

- **Be honest with yourself.** How do you react to the picture your wheel shows? What are some things that might be holding you back in an area?
- **Go with your gut.** Several areas might need more attention. You don't have to work on all of them at once. Follow your instinct—the one that's screaming "Pick me first!"
- **Plan and prepare.** Paying attention to neglected areas means committing time to them. Create a plan you can stick to.
- **Get support.** A professional can help in areas like health and finances. Consider also asking loved ones, friends, or colleagues.
- **Balance.** Is the area that's going best the thing you spend the most time on? Is it holding you back in others? Putting too much effort into any one area can throw you off balance.
- **Have fun.** If working to balance your life feels burdensome, consider taking a step back. How might you build some enjoyment into each area?

Pursuits and passions

Think back to before your addictive behavior started taking up a lot of your time. You probably enjoyed a few hobbies and activities and wanted to try others. Maybe there was something you loved to do when you were younger but got distracted from. Now's the time to bring those interests back or explore new ones.

We're talking about finding long-term activities that sustain your interest. "Hobbies" doesn't quite capture it. Instead, these are pursuits or passions that can help bring the pleasure of living back into your life.

If nothing jumps out right away, look back at your cost-benefit analysis. What benefits were you getting from your addictive behavior before the costs outweighed them? Did you enjoy the buzz? Perhaps mountain biking, horror movies, or participating in an open mic night. Did you like being able to just check out for a bit? Consider solitary road trips, hikes, or reading fiction. Was it the taste, or having the attention of others? Each one-time benefit is a clue that can guide you toward a pursuit that satisfies you.

You don't have to choose just one. Find passions and pursuits and keep looking for more. The only caution is to revisit your lifestyle balance wheel periodically: You don't want your new passion to throw off the balance you've achieved.

Tool 6.2: Explore new pursuits and passions

(vital absorbing creative interests)

Date:

Jot down pursuits that interest you. Rate each by how much you expect to enjoy it. Once you've had a chance to try it, rate it again. What surprises you?

Pursuit	**Expectation (1-10)**	**Reality (1-10)**	**Comments/thoughts**

More copies on page 87

Lifestyle goals

Look back at your lifestyle balance wheel (page 72). What areas of your life could use some attention? One may be regaining your physical, mental, and emotional health. Another may be rediscovering passions and interests.

Putting it all together requires planning, flexibility, creativity, and energy. Setting goals is a great way to start. It's a skill we tend to let weaken when we're focused on immediate satisfaction. Goals help you set priorities and point your new life in the direction you want it to go. And they're most meaningful when they connect to your values (page 29).

Where to start

Consider starting with a few short-term goals. You can set long-term goals once you have some practice.

Common goal areas	
Finances	Save money Pay off bills Donate to charity
Friends and family	Improve relationships Make new friends Spend time with kids
Career	Find a new job Build skills toward promotion Make a career transition
Physical health	Rebuild muscle Get more steps per day Eat differently Get more sleep
Passions	Pick up a new hobby Grow skills at an art form
Education	Finish your degree Take classes for fun Improve job prospects
Volunteering	Get more involved with SMART Help at a hospital or school Work at an animal shelter
Social activities	Dancing classes Book clubs Church groups

Setting effective goals

One pitfall can be setting too many goals. You want to make them realistic, but not uninteresting. Good goals are SMART (nope, no relation!):

- **Specific.** Instead of "improve my health," plan to "run a marathon" or "decrease my cholesterol."
- **Measurable.** "Go to bed by 10 p.m." is stronger than just "get more sleep."
- **Agreeable.** Choose something you like, of course. Make your goal something you want to do, not something you only think you should do.
- **Realistic.** If you've never run a marathon before, start with a 5k.
- **Time-bound.** Give yourself an end date if you can. Are you giving yourself a week to accomplish it? A year?

Here's an example of a goal that isn't a SMART goal. While it's agreeable and realistic, it is not specific, measurable, or time bound.

Goal: Eat better.				
Specific	Measurable	Agreeable	Realistic	Time-bound
		✓	✓	

Here's how that goal might be changed to improve its usefulness:

Goal: Eat more heart-healthy foods to lower my cholesterol below 200 mg/dL within 6 months.				
Specific	Measurable	Agreeable	Realistic	Time-bound
✓	✓	✓	✓	✓

When you have a good goal, then you can break it into steps:

Tasks to reach my goal:
Eat red meat 1x/month. No hamburgers or bacon. Eat fish 3x/week. Tuna sandwiches 2x/week. 1 healthy new fish recipe for dinner. Follow doctor's recommendations and get regular cholesterol tests.

Here's another example with both aspects filled in:

Goal: Show up for all visitation sessions with my kids on time for the next 3 months.				
Specific	Measurable	Agreeable	Realistic	Time-bound
✓	✓	✓	✓	✓
Tasks to reach my goal: Create an electronic calendar with reminders for visitation sessions from March to May. Leave 1 hour before session to be on time. Talk to boss on Wednesday to schedule time off I need to make sessions.				

Tool 6.3: Set an effective goal				
Goal:				
Specific	Measurable	Agreeable	Realistic	Time-bound
Tasks to reach my goal:				
More copies on page 89				

Goal tips

- Align your goals with spokes that needed attention in your lifestyle balance wheel (page 72).
- Don't set so many goals that you get overwhelmed.
- Add weekly to-dos where you can see them. Set electronic reminders if it makes sense.
- Check off tasks you finish. If you miss one, move it to the next week.
- If you're postponing tasks over and over, think about fine-tuning your goal.
- Keep a list of completed tasks to remind you of the progress you've made.

Maintaining a healthy mind

Meditation and relaxation are different for everyone, so it's important to find what works best for you. This might include progressive muscle relaxation, mindful breathing, visualization, or listening to calming sounds. For those with limitations, some of the exercises presented here may be difficult or impossible. We encourage you to explore and discover methods that help you find a sense of calm and balance regardless of your ability.

Mindfulness and meditation

Strong emotions are inevitable, as we discussed in Chapter 5. Awareness techniques like meditation can help you maintain your balance. Many people ruminate or return to cycles of unhelpful thoughts. Others feel easily caught up in uncomfortable feelings or urges.

Mindfulness is learning to pay attention to the present moment. It's the opposite of mindlessness. It describes a state of active, nonjudgmental attention to the present.

Research into mindfulness shows it reduces depression, obsessive thinking, stress, anger, and even post-traumatic stress. Evidence suggests it helps people in overcoming addictive behaviors.

A simple meditation is one way to integrate mindfulness into your day. It does take practice. At first, you may only be able to meditate for a few minutes, but the more you do it, the longer you'll be able to do it. Some days it'll be easier than others. It helps if you do it at the same time and same place every day.

Tool 6.4: Meditation practice

Date:

Set a timer—five minutes is plenty to start. Sit in a comfortable upright posture with a straight back. Don't make yourself feel rigid, but don't slouch. (Slouching affects your breathing, an important part of meditation.)

Some people sit on pillows in the Buddhist lotus position. For this, tuck your ankles under you and rest your hands on your knees, palms up. Others sit in a comfortable chair. You may want to burn a candle or incense. Meditative music may help, too. Experiment to find what works best for you.

Breathe slowly through your nose and fill your lungs. Notice how your belly expands and sticks out when you breathe in. Put your hands there to feel it.

Close your eyes. Take three deep, long breaths, noticing how it feels.

Now, let your breath settle to a normal rhythm. On the out-breath, silently count "one." On the next out-breath, count "two." Keep going up to ten. When you get to ten, go back to one. If you lose count, just start again at one.

Feel the physical sensation of your breathing. Thoughts will enter your mind. Don't try to push them away or pretend they don't exist. Recognize their presence but don't engage them. If your mind wanders, gently turn your attention back to your breathing and counting. Don't judge yourself or your meditation "abilities."

Do this until your timer runs out. Pay attention to the present and those excessive emotions. Over time, ruminating and troublesome thoughts may trouble you less.

You also can practice being mindful wherever you are. Just notice what you feel and think wherever you are. Maybe it's the feeling of the breeze or the presence of another person. The only requirement is taking time to be aware of the world around and within you.

Some people get frustrated because they can't "turn off their thoughts" while meditating and assume they're not doing it right. In reality, you can't prevent thoughts from popping up. It's common during practice for your mind to wander. The essence of meditation is to learn to notice and acknowledge these thoughts and then return to your breath or chosen anchor.

Relaxation

Learning to relax may seem like a luxury or a self-indulgence, but it helps restore balance to your life. Although they're similar, meditation and relaxation aren't the same.

Relaxation is different for everyone, so find what works for you. Progressive muscle relaxation is one technique you can try. The goal is to become aware of how your muscles feel when they're tense versus relaxed. Many people report feeling immediately refreshed. You may feel this way, or you may feel nothing.

Tool 6.5: Progressive muscle relaxation practice

Date:

You can do this lying down or in a chair. Tense each muscle group and hold it for five seconds. Then relax instantly for 10 seconds or more. Compare how each one feels before and after. Don't tense any muscle group that is a problem for you.

Head	Wrinkle your forehead Close your eyes tightly Open your mouth wide Push your tongue against the roof of your mouth
Neck and shoulders	Shrug your shoulders toward your ears Press your shoulder blades together
Arms and hands	Clench your hands into fists Curl your biceps in toward your chest Extend your arms straight, and push against an invisible wall.
Stomach, lower back, hips, and butt	Tighten your stomach muscles Arch your back Tighten your hip and butt muscles
Legs	Squeeze your thighs together Tense your calf muscles
Ankles and feet	Flex your ankles, bringing your toes up Point your feet and toes Curl your toes under

There are many variations to this experience. You can do one side of your body at a time. You can focus on the muscle group without tensing it. You can do each group several times before going to the next. Do what works best for you. This experience could take 10 minutes, or 30 minutes or longer. Accept whatever thoughts or images arise but keep returning your attention to your muscles. This experience is sometimes easier for people than meditation because of the muscle activity.

Visualization

Our imagination is more powerful than we realize. We'll focus on visualization for relaxation. But know that it can help you prepare for job interviews, hard conversations, and even your goals. Athletes use visualization to enhance their performance. Public speakers often visualize going through their presentations before giving them.

For this relaxation exercise, allow yourself about 15 minutes. Make sure you don't feel rushed and prevent distractions if you can. Sit or lie down in a comfortable, quiet place.

Tool 6.6: Visualization practice

Date:

Close your eyes. See yourself entering a quiet, safe, and relaxing place alone. Fill your place with details of what you hear and smell. Imagine what you're sitting or lying on, or how you might be moving around. Create in your mind the noises and smells that you find relaxing.

Fill this place with as much detail as you can about things that relax you. Let your body relax and your shoulders and head fall gently.

Breathe slowly.

Regaining your health

Nutrition

Healthy, balanced eating is important. How and where you eat depends on your situation. Eating at home can involve making shopping lists, purchasing groceries, prepping meals and cleaning up. Going out for an occasional meal can be fun. However, meals at home can be more nutritious than meals out. Make a shopping list, get groceries, prep your meals, and clean up. These activities can also help fill time and enhance relationships at home.

For a variety of reasons, vitamin deficiencies are common in many who've experienced addictive behaviors. For example: Heavy alcohol use flushes your body of water-soluble vitamins. These include B vitamins (such as thiamine and folic acid) and vitamin C. You might choose to consult with a qualified health professional to get guidance about possible vitamin supplements.

Exercise

Any form of physical exercise is beneficial. You don't have to join a gym or lift weights or do brisk aerobics unless you feel fit enough. Don't underestimate the power of regular walks or bike rides. Exercise doesn't have to be strenuous to be beneficial. Evidence suggests that 30-minute walks five days a week can reverse the effects of depression, if you can work up to that. But any exercise is helpful, and a quick exercise break in your day can help you feel more positive and productive.

If you haven't exercised regularly, build up gradually. Consider balancing your activities across aerobics, strength, balance, and stretching. If you have any reservations about your health, check with a health professional before you get started.

Sleep

Sleep is a third major factor in healthy living. Many of us would benefit from more sleep. Expect your sleep patterns to change as your daily routine evolves. Your body is adjusting! Cutting down on caffeine, taking a short walk in the evening, or reading a book in bed may help to improve your sleep.

It may take weeks to recover from a sleep deficit and to start sleeping normally. Vivid, sometimes disturbing dreams are common early in recovery. It takes some time for sleep patterns to improve. If your sleep does not seem to be improving quickly enough, you could consult with a qualified health professional or search for information about "sleep hygiene," a term for improving your sleep habits.

Medication

SMART supports the informed use of qualified psychological treatment and prescribed medications. The use of medications is a highly personal decision which should not be debated in SMART meetings. Always consult with a qualified health professional before reducing or ending use of a medication.

Procrastination

Procrastination is a universal, and sometimes useful, human behavior. Like anything, it can cause harm if it becomes extreme. You can apply what you've learned about addictive behavior to procrastination too.

A few points to keep in mind:

- Procrastination can weaken your ability to achieve your goals.
- It can be a form of self-sabotage.
- It can be associated with trying to avoid uncomfortable emotions like anxiety.
- It might be a signal that you're not sure how you feel.

The tools in Chapter 5 may be useful when working through why you are procrastinating and how to change.

Summary

Living a balanced life can be exhilarating and authentic.

- This is your life, and you get to choose how to live it.
- You can experiment with different aspects of your life to determine what adds value and balance.
- Setting goals, planning tasks, and developing passions and pursuits can help you feel fulfilled.
- SMART activities and meetings are available whenever you want.
- Consider becoming a meeting facilitator when you feel like it would contribute to your balanced life.
- The tools you practice in SMART can prove valuable in life, not just in your current change process.

Chapter 7: Putting it all together

SMART's foundation is self-empowerment, science, progress, and the whole person. On these principles, we provide general ideas about the process of change. This handbook is filled with tools we believe could be helpful to you.

In SMART we recognize that we share much in common, and some of our experiences are unique. For example, traumatic experiences may affect you in ways you don't understand. You may have genetic predispositions to developing an addictive behavior based on the challenges of your ancestors! You may have significant sensory sensitivities. Some of these things can be worked on with the help of mental health professionals. Others are outside of your control.

You might visualize this as follows: We're all doing our best to live balanced lives. For some of us, that balancing act occurs on the tip of a triangle because of significant factors out of our control.

For others, living a balanced life takes a bit less work because of a different set of factors.

Regardless, you can decide how you'd like to improve the stability of the platform on which you balance your life. You get to decide what internal practices and external supports are helpful for you.

Your chosen supports may include SMART meetings, and they may not. Regardless, we will be here to support you if you decide to join a meeting.

Embracing "and"

As you continue your journey, consider one change that may be helpful – the power of "and." The idea that two statements can be true at the same time is at the heart of dialectical behavior therapy (DBT). You can practice this by noticing the word "but" in your thoughts and replacing it with the word "and."

Here are some examples:

- I feel sad **and** I know that my feelings are not permanent.
- I am experiencing discomfort, **and** I have a tool I can use to surf it.
- I want to drink, **and** I have other choices available to me.
- I am angry at my parent, **and** I want to maintain a relationship with them.

Notice how different these statements sound than if they contained the word "but." Everything before a "but" feels minimized or dismissed. Give this a try as you continue to practice what you've learned.

The power of choice

For some people, the responsibility of making decisions about change can feel like too much. They want more specific guidance. Other approaches are available, and they can be effective. Most approaches to change require effort, but the self-empowering approach also requires making decisions and learning to trust yourself. SMART does not push you into a one-size-fits-all approach. Even if it doesn't feel like it all the time, you are the expert on your life.

Fortunately, not all decisions need to be made at once. Some decisions can be broken down into smaller ones. Often you can start with small steps and learn that you have the power of choice.

You are always welcome to try other approaches instead of or alongside ours. Or do whatever you think is best for the changes you want to make. There are as many pathways to change as there are individuals. The best recovery approach is the one that works for you. You get to decide what that approach is.

Finally, we encourage you to try attending SMART meetings if you haven't already. Talk about your experiences, keep a journal, and read more about topics that come up and issues that concern you. See if attending the same groups week to week helps you open up to yourself with the support of others.

However you decide to proceed, we wish you the best!

Tool quick reference guide

This table maps the SMART tools to the Stages of Change. It can help you identify which ones are most helpful at each stage.

Tool	Page	Precontemplation	Contemplation	Preparation	Action	Maintenance
2.1 Journaling	23	X	X	X	X	X
2.2 Practice self-compassion	24	X	X	X	X	X
3.1 Cost Benefit Analysis	26		X	X		
3.2 Define your values (hierarchy of values)	29	X	X	X		
3.3 Five questions	30		X	X		
3.4 Create a change plan	31		X	X	X	X
4.1 Identify triggers	38			X	X	
4.2 Rank trigger risks	39			X	X	
4.3 Log your urges	40			X	X	
4.4 Plan your week	45				X	X
4.5 Customize DENTS for you	46				X	X
4.6 Personify and disarm	48				X	
5.1 Dispute unhelpful beliefs	56				X	X
5.2 ABC exercise	61				X	X
5.3 Practice problem solving	64			X	X	X
5.4 Planning positive conversations	66		X	X	X	X
5.5 Setting healthy boundaries	68		X	X	X	X
6.1 Check your lifestyle balance (lifestyle balance wheel)	72			X	X	X
6.2 Explore new passions and pursuits	75			X	X	X
6.3 Set an effective goal	79			X	X	X
6.4 Meditation practice	80				X	X
6.5 Try progressive muscle relaxation	82				X	X
6.6 Visualize a relaxing space	83				X	X

Sources

Cameron, J. (2002). **The artist's way: A spiritual path to higher creativity.** TarcherPerigee.

Ellis, A., & Harper, R. A. (1989). **A new guide to rational living.** Wilshire Book Co.

Horvath, A. T. (2004). **Sex, drugs, gambling, and chocolate: A workbook for overcoming addictions.** Impact.

Liese, B. S., & Beck, A. T. (2022). **Cognitive behavioral therapy of addictive behaviors.** The Guilford Press.

Neff, K. (2011). **Self-compassion: Stop Beating Yourself Up and Leave Insecurity Behind.** William Morrow.

Acknowledgments

On behalf of this edition's editor, Louisa Diomalli, we extend a special thanks to: Pete Rubinas, Tom Horvath, David Koss, Melina Gilbert, Alison Beck, Louis Leake, Amanda Clearwater, Eboni Jewel Sears, Roxanne Allen, Sandy Dickson, Antoinette Gavel-Ouellette, Tammy Ginader, Bill Greer, Megan Goodrich, Gus Curran, Brad Glaser, and Shawn Thomas. Each donated time, insight, and candid impressions to this edition of the SMART 4-Point Handbook.

ADDITIONAL COPIES OF TOOL SHEETS

Visit the SMART Recovery website to download additional copies.

Tool 2.2: Practice self-compassion

Self-compassion is a practice that can help address feelings of sadness or hopelessness. These feelings are common when working to address an addictive behavior One model of self-compassion defines it as a practice comprised of these three things:

- Being kind to yourself rather than judging yourself
- Recognizing that what you struggle with is something that you have in common with other humans
- Practicing mindfulness rather than over-identifying with your thoughts and emotions.

How can you practice these three things in your life? Jot some ideas down below. Pick one at a time to practice until they become habitual. With practice, you may find that self-compassion arises more quickly and with less effort, helping you stay present in each moment and reducing your stress.

Self-kindness practices	Common humanity practice	Mindfulness practice
Ex: Ask myself if that's how I would talk to a friend in this situation, stop calling myself names	Ex: Attend mutual support group meetings, volunteer	Ex: Daily meditation; notice the birds I hear on a walk

Tool 2.2: Practice self-compassion

Self-compassion is a practice that can help address feelings of sadness or hopelessness. These feelings are common when working to address an addictive behavior One model of self-compassion defines it as a practice comprised of these three things:

- Being kind to yourself rather than judging yourself
- Recognizing that what you struggle with is something that you have in common with other humans
- Practicing mindfulness rather than over-identifying with your thoughts and emotions.

How can you practice these three things in your life? Jot some ideas down below. Pick one at a time to practice until they become habitual. With practice, you may find that self-compassion arises more quickly and with less effort, helping you stay present in each moment and reducing your stress.

Self-kindness practices	Common humanity practice	Mindfulness practice
Ex: Ask myself if that's how I would talk to a friend in this situation, stop calling myself names	Ex: Attend mutual support group meetings, volunteer	Ex: Daily meditation; notice the birds I hear on a walk

Tool 2.2: Practice self-compassion

Self-compassion is a practice that can help address feelings of sadness or hopelessness. These feelings are common when working to address an addictive behavior One model of self-compassion defines it as a practice comprised of these three things:

- Being kind to yourself rather than judging yourself
- Recognizing that what you struggle with is something that you have in common with other humans
- Practicing mindfulness rather than over-identifying with your thoughts and emotions.

How can you practice these three things in your life? Jot some ideas down below. Pick one at a time to practice until they become habitual. With practice, you may find that self-compassion arises more quickly and with less effort, helping you stay present in each moment and reducing your stress.

Self-kindness practices	Common humanity practice	Mindfulness practice
Ex: Ask myself if that's how I would talk to a friend in this situation, stop calling myself names	Ex: Attend mutual support group meetings, volunteer	Ex: Daily meditation; notice the birds I hear on a walk

Tool 3.1: Cost-benefit analysis

You get something out of the behavior you're thinking about changing. Otherwise, you wouldn't have engaged in it. Consciously or otherwise, at some point you decided the benefits outweighed the costs. Do they now?

It's normal to both want to change and not want to change. It's also difficult to hold the short- and long-term benefits and costs of a behavior in one's awareness at the same time. This tool can help with these challenges.

Write your benefits and costs in the boxes below. See page 27 for some questions to get you started.

The behavior I'm analyzing:

Today's date:

When I do this behavior

Benefits (rewards or advantages)	**Costs (risks and disadvantages)**
Ex: I feel more alert, I don't feel pain, I feel more attractive	Ex: Hangovers, losing my partner's trust*, hard to pay my bills on time

When I don't do this behavior

Benefits (rewards or advantages)	**Costs (risks and disadvantages)**
Ex: Save money*, do better at work	Ex: Feel stressed, body aches

After you make your lists, star the long-term benefits and costs. Where are you sacrificing your future goals for immediate satisfaction in the present?

Tool 3.1: Cost-benefit analysis

You get something out of the behavior you're thinking about changing. Otherwise, you wouldn't have engaged in it. Consciously or otherwise, at some point you decided the benefits outweighed the costs. Do they now?

It's normal to both want to change and not want to change. It's also difficult to hold the short- and long-term benefits and costs of a behavior in one's awareness at the same time. This tool can help with these challenges.

Write your benefits and costs in the boxes below. See page 27 for some questions to get you started.

The behavior I'm analyzing:

Today's date:

When I do this behavior

Benefits (rewards or advantages)	**Costs (risks and disadvantages)**
Ex: I feel more alert, I don't feel pain, I feel more attractive	Ex: Hangovers, losing my partner's trust*, hard to pay my bills on time

When I don't do this behavior

Benefits (rewards or advantages)	**Costs (risks and disadvantages)**
Ex: Save money*, do better at work	Ex: Feel stressed, body aches

After you make your lists, star the long-term benefits and costs. Where are you sacrificing your future goals for immediate satisfaction in the present?

Tool 3.1: Cost-benefit analysis

You get something out of the behavior you're thinking about changing. Otherwise, you wouldn't have engaged in it. Consciously or otherwise, at some point you decided the benefits outweighed the costs. Do they now?

It's normal to both want to change and not want to change. It's also difficult to hold the short- and long-term benefits and costs of a behavior in one's awareness at the same time. This tool can help with these challenges.

Write your benefits and costs in the boxes below. See page 27 for some questions to get you started.

The behavior I'm analyzing:

Today's date:

When I do this behavior

Benefits (rewards or advantages) Ex: I feel more alert, I don't feel pain, I feel more attractive	**Costs (risks and disadvantages)** Ex: Hangovers, losing my partner's trust*, hard to pay my bills on time

When I don't do this behavior

Benefits (rewards or advantages) Ex: Save money*, do better at work	**Costs (risks and disadvantages)** Ex: Feel stressed, body aches

After you make your lists, star the long-term benefits and costs. Where are you sacrificing your future goals for immediate satisfaction in the present?

Tool 3.2: Define your values (hierarchy of values)

We all have values in life. And although they underpin all our feelings and decisions, we rarely think about them explicitly. Examining them and writing them down can help you focus on what matters most.

Start by jotting down as many of your values as you can—anything that you think matters to you. There are no right or wrong answers. Some examples: financial independence, my family, honesty, being happy, the environment, travel, solitude, or my health.

Next, go back and circle the big ones, or group your notes into themes. Ultimately, try to narrow your list to your top five.

My values
1.
2.
3.
4.
5.

What actions align with your values?

Now, look over your list. For most people, the behavior they want to change isn't a value. Yet it may have made itself a priority in your life. Where does your behavior conflict with your value system?

Notes:

Tool 3.2: Define your values (hierarchy of values)

We all have values in life. And although they underpin all our feelings and decisions, we rarely think about them explicitly. Examining them and writing them down can help you focus on what matters most.

Start by jotting down as many of your values as you can—anything that you think matters to you. There are no right or wrong answers. Some examples: financial independence, my family, honesty, being happy, the environment, travel, solitude, or my health.

Next, go back and circle the big ones, or group your notes into themes. Ultimately, try to narrow your list to your top five.

My values
1.
2.
3.
4.
5.

What actions align with your values?

Now, look over your list. For most people, the behavior they want to change isn't a value. Yet it may have made itself a priority in your life. Where does your behavior conflict with your value system?

Notes:

Tool 3.2: Define your values (hierarchy of values)

We all have values in life. And although they underpin all our feelings and decisions, we rarely think about them explicitly. Examining them and writing them down can help you focus on what matters most.

Start by jotting down as many of your values as you can—anything that you think matters to you. There are no right or wrong answers. Some examples: financial independence, my family, honesty, being happy, the environment, travel, solitude, or my health.

Next, go back and circle the big ones, or group your notes into themes. Ultimately, try to narrow your list to your top five.

My values
1.
2.
3.
4.
5.

What actions align with your values?

Now, look over your list. For most people, the behavior they want to change isn't a value. Yet it may have made itself a priority in your life. Where does your behavior conflict with your value system?

Notes:

Tool 3.3: Five questions about getting what I want

Sometimes it's hard to see what you could do differently to achieve your goals. Your goal in this exercise may be to reduce or resolve an addictive behavior, or it may be something broader.

1. What do I want for my future?

Examples: To get my degree, to be a good parent, to be financially independent

2. What am I doing to achieve that now?

Ex: Bookmarked ideas, talked to a friend, started an application

3. How do I feel about what I'm doing now?

Ex: Dissatisfied, stuck, guilty, stressed, disconnected

4. What could I do differently to help me get what I want?

5. How would changing what I do or getting what I want make me feel?

Compare your feelings about what you're doing (2) with how you'd feel if you changed your approach (5). Could the difference between the two motivate you? Could the activities in (4) help take the place of your addictive behavior? And if so—how much more quickly might you reach your goal in (1)?

Tool 3.3: Five questions about getting what I want

Sometimes it's hard to see what you could do differently to achieve your goals. Your goal in this exercise may be to reduce or resolve an addictive behavior, or it may be something broader.

1. What do I want for my future?

Examples: To get my degree, to be a good parent, to be financially independent

2. What am I doing to achieve that now?

Ex: Bookmarked ideas, talked to a friend, started an application

3. How do I feel about what I'm doing now?

Ex: Dissatisfied, stuck, guilty, stressed, disconnected

4. What could I do differently to help me get what I want?

5. How would changing what I do or getting what I want make me feel?

Compare your feelings about what you're doing (2) with how you'd feel if you changed your approach (5). Could the difference between the two motivate you? Could the activities in (4) help take the place of your addictive behavior? And if so—how much more quickly might you reach your goal in (1)?

Tool 3.3: Five questions about getting what I want

Sometimes it's hard to see what you could do differently to achieve your goals. Your goal in this exercise may be to reduce or resolve an addictive behavior, or it may be something broader.

1. What do I want for my future?

Examples: To get my degree, to be a good parent, to be financially independent

2. What am I doing to achieve that now?

Ex: Bookmarked ideas, talked to a friend, started an application

3. How do I feel about what I'm doing now?

Ex: Dissatisfied, stuck, guilty, stressed, disconnected

4. What could I do differently to help me get what I want?

5. How would changing what I do or getting what I want make me feel?

Compare your feelings about what you're doing (2) with how you'd feel if you changed your approach (5). Could the difference between the two motivate you? Could the activities in (4) help take the place of your addictive behavior? And if so—how much more quickly might you reach your goal in (1)?

Tool 3.4: Create a change plan

You're getting clearer about what you want for your future. Now you need a plan. Use this worksheet to identify steps you can take toward the future you envision. Consider who can help you get there. Remember that strategies are just ideas. If your first (or hundredth) plan doesn't work, try a new one.

My change plan	**Date:**
Changes I want to make: (Ex: Avoid bars/clubs, sleep better, abstain within 1 week)	
How important are these changes to me? (Rate from 1-10.)	
How confident am I that I can make these changes? (Rate from 1-10.)	
The most important reasons I want to make this change is: Ex: I want to keep my job, I want my kids back, I'm concerned about my health	
The steps I plan to take are: Ex: Attend SMART meetings, plan healthy meals each week, make a doctor's appointment	
Who can help me and how:	
Person	**Kind of help**
Ex: Friend	Share healthy recipes
I'll know my plan is working when: Ex: I can afford my own apartment, I'm always on time to work, I can have a normal conversation with my mom	
Some things that could interfere with my plan are: Ex: Having no plans on a weekend night, holiday season parties, last-minute changes to work schedule	
I'll check in with myself on this change plan on (date):	
Consider marking this date on your calendar, so you don't forget. If your plan isn't working out, edit it or start fresh and try again.	

Tool 3.4: Create a change plan

You're getting clearer about what you want for your future. Now you need a plan. Use this worksheet to identify steps you can take toward the future you envision. Consider who can help you get there. Remember that strategies are just ideas. If your first (or hundredth) plan doesn't work, try a new one.

My change plan	**Date:**
Changes I want to make: (Ex: Avoid bars/clubs, sleep better, abstain within 1 week)	
How important are these changes to me? (Rate from 1-10.)	
How confident am I that I can make these changes? (Rate from 1-10.)	
The most important reasons I want to make this change is: Ex: I want to keep my job, I want my kids back, I'm concerned about my health	
The steps I plan to take are: Ex: Attend SMART meetings, plan healthy meals each week, make a doctor's appointment	
Who can help me and how:	
Person	**Kind of help**
Ex: Friend	Share healthy recipes
I'll know my plan is working when: Ex: I can afford my own apartment, I'm always on time to work, I can have a normal conversation with my mom	
Some things that could interfere with my plan are: Ex: Having no plans on a weekend night, holiday season parties, last-minute changes to work schedule	
I'll check in with myself on this change plan on (date):	
Consider marking this date on your calendar, so you don't forget. If your plan isn't working out, edit it or start fresh and try again.	

Tool 3.4: Create a change plan

You're getting clearer about what you want for your future. Now you need a plan. Use this worksheet to identify steps you can take toward the future you envision. Consider who can help you get there. Remember that strategies are just ideas. If your first (or hundredth) plan doesn't work, try a new one.

My change plan	**Date:**
Changes I want to make: (Ex: Avoid bars/clubs, sleep better, abstain within 1 week)	
How important are these changes to me? (Rate from 1-10.)	
How confident am I that I can make these changes? (Rate from 1-10.)	
The most important reasons I want to make this change is: Ex: I want to keep my job, I want my kids back, I'm concerned about my health	
The steps I plan to take are: Ex: Attend SMART meetings, plan healthy meals each week, make a doctor's appointment	
Who can help me and how:	
Person	**Kind of help**
Ex: Friend	Share healthy recipes
I'll know my plan is working when: Ex: I can afford my own apartment, I'm always on time to work, I can have a normal conversation with my mom	
Some things that could interfere with my plan are: Ex: Having no plans on a weekend night, holiday season parties, last-minute changes to work schedule	
I'll check in with myself on this change plan on (date):	
Consider marking this date on your calendar, so you don't forget. If your plan isn't working out, edit it or start fresh and try again.	

Tool 4.1: Identify triggers

Date:

To identify your triggers, consider each sense: sight, hearing, smell, taste, and touch. You might be surprised at how many there are. Be honest and list them all—even if they seem insignificant. If there's more than one behavior you want to change, list them all in the left column.

Behavior	**Triggers**
Ex: Gambling	Lottery ads; scratch-off tickets in stores
Ex: Drinking alcohol	Attending a wedding; Being offered a free beer at the end of a 5k run

Tool 4.1: Identify triggers

Date:

To identify your triggers, consider each sense: sight, hearing, smell, taste, and touch. You might be surprised at how many there are. Be honest and list them all—even if they seem insignificant. If there's more than one behavior you want to change, list them all in the left column.

Behavior	**Triggers**
Ex: Gambling	Lottery ads; scratch-off tickets in stores
Ex: Drinking alcohol	Attending a wedding; Being offered a free beer at the end of a 5k run

Tool 4.1: Identify triggers

Date:

To identify your triggers, consider each sense: sight, hearing, smell, taste, and touch. You might be surprised at how many there are. Be honest and list them all—even if they seem insignificant. If there's more than one behavior you want to change, list them all in the left column.

Behavior	**Triggers**
Ex: Gambling	Lottery ads; scratch-off tickets in stores
Ex: Drinking alcohol	Attending a wedding; Being offered a free beer at the end of a 5k run

Tool 4.2: Rank trigger risks

Date:

Not all triggers are equally powerful. Some are uniquely more likely to create an urge for you than others. Rate each trigger from 1 (weakest) to 10 (riskiest). Then, you can prioritize the triggers you most need to be prepared for. Key categories are listed below. Add your own from Tool 4.1.

Trigger	**Rating (1-10)**
Unpleasant emotions (ex: anger, frustration, grief) Others:	
Pleasant emotions (ex: joy, peace, anticipation) Others:	
Physical sensations (ex: pain, cold, heat) Others:	
Stress (ex: deadlines, anxiety, financial concerns) Others:	
Conflicts with others (ex: coworker, partner, family) Others:	
Places and times (ex: restaurants, cars, summer, weekends) Others:	
Other:	
Other:	
Other:	
Other:	

Tool 4.2: Rank trigger risks

Date:

Not all triggers are equally powerful. Some are uniquely more likely to create an urge for you than others. Rate each trigger from 1 (weakest) to 10 (riskiest). Then, you can prioritize the triggers you most need to be prepared for. Key categories are listed below. Add your own from Tool 4.1.

Trigger	**Rating (1-10)**
Unpleasant emotions (ex: anger, frustration, grief) Others:	
Pleasant emotions (ex: joy, peace, anticipation) Others:	
Physical sensations (ex: pain, cold, heat) Others:	
Stress (ex: deadlines, anxiety, financial concerns) Others:	
Conflicts with others (ex: coworker, partner, family) Others:	
Places and times (ex: restaurants, cars, summer, weekends) Others:	
Other:	
Other:	
Other:	
Other:	

Tool 4.2: Rank trigger risks

Date:

Not all triggers are equally powerful. Some are uniquely more likely to create an urge for you than others. Rate each trigger from 1 (weakest) to 10 (riskiest). Then, you can prioritize the triggers you most need to be prepared for. Key categories are listed below. Add your own from Tool 4.1.

Trigger	Rating (1-10)
Unpleasant emotions (ex: anger, frustration, grief) Others:	
Pleasant emotions (ex: joy, peace, anticipation) Others:	
Physical sensations (ex: pain, cold, heat) Others:	
Stress (ex: deadlines, anxiety, financial concerns) Others:	
Conflicts with others (ex: coworker, partner, family) Others:	
Places and times (ex: restaurants, cars, summer, weekends) Others:	
Other:	
Other:	
Other:	
Other:	

Tool 4.3: Log your urges

Date:

Do you know how long your urges last? Or when they're strongest? By writing them down, you'll begin to see patterns.
If you keep a journal, you can keep it with you and record your urges there. At first, you might jot down many urges per day—that's normal.

Date	Time	Strength (1-10)	Length of Urge	What triggered my urge?	Who/where was involved?	How I coped and felt about it	Ideas for next time
8/29	1:15 pm	8	1 minute	Lunch in a wine bar	Lisa and Stephanie	Told them and forgot pretty fast	Find a new lunch spot

Reflecting on your urges, what hidden triggers do you identify? Do any recurring thought patterns emerge? What places, people, or activities can you avoid or distract yourself from?

Tool 4.3: Log your urges

Date:

Do you know how long your urges last? Or when they're strongest? By writing them down, you'll begin to see patterns.
If you keep a journal, you can keep it with you and record your urges there. At first, you might jot down many urges per day—that's normal.

Date	Time	Strength (1-10)	Length of Urge	What triggered my urge?	Who/where was involved?	How I coped and felt about it	Ideas for next time
8/29	1:15 pm	8	1 minute	Lunch in a wine bar	Lisa and Stephanie	Told them and forgot pretty fast	Find a new lunch spot

Reflecting on your urges, what hidden triggers do you identify? Do any recurring thought patterns emerge? What places, people, or activities can you avoid or distract yourself from?

Tool 4.3: Log your urges

Date:

Do you know how long your urges last? Or when they're strongest? By writing them down, you'll begin to see patterns.
If you keep a journal, you can keep it with you and record your urges there. At first, you might jot down many urges per day—that's normal.

Date	Time	Strength (1-10)	Length of Urge	What triggered my urge?	Who/where was involved?	How I coped and felt about it	Ideas for next time
8/29	1:15 pm	8	1 minute	Lunch in a wine bar	Lisa and Stephanie	Told them and forgot pretty fast	Find a new lunch spot

Reflecting on your urges, what hidden triggers do you identify? Do any recurring thought patterns emerge? What places, people, or activities can you avoid or distract yourself from?

Tool 4.4: Plan your week

Sometimes having a plan for your week can help you avoid triggering situations. Try adding healthy distractions and activities throughout your week.

Time	Monday	Tuesday	Wednesday	Thursday	Friday	Saturday	Sunday
Morning							
Midday							
Evening							

Tool 4.4: Plan your week

Sometimes having a plan for your week can help you avoid triggering situations. Try adding healthy distractions and activities throughout your week.

Time	Monday	Tuesday	Wednesday	Thursday	Friday	Saturday	Sunday
Morning							
Midday							
Evening							

Tool 4.4: Plan your week

Sometimes having a plan for your week can help you avoid triggering situations. Try adding healthy distractions and activities throughout your week.

Time	Monday	Tuesday	Wednesday	Thursday	Friday	Saturday	Sunday
Morning							
Midday							
Evening							

Tool 4.5: Customize DENTS for you

DENTS (page 46) can help you remember how to get through an urge. Once you're familiar with it, write down what strategies help you in each row.

Deny or delay	How long do urges last if you don't give in? How bad do they get before they fade?
Escape	What triggers can you get away from? How can you minimize their influence?
Neutralize	What techniques help you sit with urges until they pass? What words or SMART activities provide comfort?
Tasks	What activities absorb you fully enough to fend off urges?
Swap	What positive thoughts chase out your negative ones during an urge? What healthy activities clear your mind?

Tool 4.5: Customize DENTS for you

DENTS (page 46) can help you remember how to get through an urge. Once you're familiar with it, write down what strategies help you in each row.

Deny or delay	How long do urges last if you don't give in? How bad do they get before they fade?
Escape	What triggers can you get away from? How can you minimize their influence?
Neutralize	What techniques help you sit with urges until they pass? What words or SMART activities provide comfort?
Tasks	What activities absorb you fully enough to fend off urges?
Swap	What positive thoughts chase out your negative ones during an urge? What healthy activities clear your mind?

Tool 4.5: Customize DENTS for you

DENTS (page 46) can help you remember how to get through an urge. Once you're familiar with it, write down what strategies help you in each row.

Deny or delay	How long do urges last if you don't give in? How bad do they get before they fade?
Escape	What triggers can you get away from? How can you minimize their influence?
Neutralize	What techniques help you sit with urges until they pass? What words or SMART activities provide comfort?
Tasks	What activities absorb you fully enough to fend off urges?
Swap	What positive thoughts chase out your negative ones during an urge? What healthy activities clear your mind?

Tool 4.6: Personify and disarm

Date:	
The urges you feel aren't you. They're an impulse or a reaction—something separate from you. For some, personifying urges can create a helpful boundary. It also helps something abstract feel more concrete and manageable.	
Name	Ex: The whiner, the lobbyist, the hurt child
What you say or do to them	Ex: I see you and I am in control here; I hear you and don't need your help anymore.
What happens when you say it	Ex: They lose their power, they dissolve, they move on

Tool 4.6: Personify and disarm

Date:	
The urges you feel aren't you. They're an impulse or a reaction—something separate from you. For some, personifying urges can create a helpful boundary. It also helps something abstract feel more concrete and manageable.	
Name	Ex: The whiner, the lobbyist, the hurt child
What you say or do to them	Ex: I see you and I am in control here; I hear you and don't need your help anymore.
What happens when you say it	Ex: They lose their power, they dissolve, they move on

Tool 4.6: Personify and disarm

Date:	
The urges you feel aren't you. They're an impulse or a reaction—something separate from you. For some, personifying urges can create a helpful boundary. It also helps something abstract feel more concrete and manageable.	
Name	Ex: The whiner, the lobbyist, the hurt child
What you say or do to them	Ex: I see you and I am in control here; I hear you and don't need your help anymore.
What happens when you say it	Ex: They lose their power, they dissolve, they move on

Tool 5.1: Dispute unhelpful beliefs

Date:

Refer to the table of common unhelpful beliefs (page 54) or write down your own. Then, question the belief and provide a more reasonable alternative.

My unhelpful belief	Question	Helpful belief
Ex: I can't deal with this without using.	Can I deal with it?	It might be hard, but I can. It's going to get easier.

Tool 5.1: Dispute unhelpful beliefs

Date:

Refer to the table of common unhelpful beliefs (page 54) or write down your own. Then, question the belief and provide a more reasonable alternative.

My unhelpful belief	Question	Helpful belief
Ex: I can't deal with this without using.	Can I deal with it?	It might be hard, but I can. It's going to get easier.

Tool 5.1: Dispute unhelpful beliefs

Date:

Refer to the table of common unhelpful beliefs (page 54) or write down your own. Then, question the belief and provide a more reasonable alternative.

My unhelpful belief	Question	Helpful belief
Ex: I can't deal with this without using.	Can I deal with it?	It might be hard, but I can. It's going to get easier.

Tool 5.2: ABC exercise

Date:

Activating event	**Belief about the event**	**Consequence of the unhelpful belief**	**Dispute the unhelpful belief**	**Effective thinking change**
The event that created the urge.	What I unhelpfully believe about A—the "must."	How I feel and behave in response to A because of B.	Questions I ask myself to dispute the unhelpful belief B	The new more effective belief I adopt to replace B, which leads to a different C in response to A.
Ex: My boss yelled at me today in front of my coworkers.	He has no right to embarrass me. It's not fair. I can't stand this.	I'm really mad and I want a drink.	Does my boss only yell at me? Is life always fair? Can I stand this without a drink?	My boss yells at everyone sooner or later. Life isn't fair. That didn't feel great, and it's over. My boss isn't worth giving up my long-term goals.

Tool 5.2: ABC exercise

Date:

Activating event	Belief about the event	Consequence of the unhelpful belief	Dispute the unhelpful belief	Effective thinking change
The event that created the urge.	What I unhelpfully believe about A—the "must."	How I feel and behave in response to A because of B.	Questions I ask myself to dispute the unhelpful belief B	The new more effective belief I adopt to replace B, which leads to a different C in response to A.
Ex: My boss yelled at me today in front of my coworkers.	He has no right to embarrass me. It's not fair. I can't stand this.	I'm really mad and I want a drink.	Does my boss only yell at me? Is life always fair? Can I stand this without a drink?	My boss yells at everyone sooner or later. Life isn't fair. That didn't feel great, and it's over. My boss isn't worth giving up my long-term goals.

Tool 5.2: ABC exercise

Date:

Activating event	**Belief about the event**	**Consequence of the unhelpful belief**	**Dispute the unhelpful belief**	**Effective thinking change**
The event that created the urge.	What I unhelpfully believe about A—the "must."	How I feel and behave in response to A because of B.	Questions I ask myself to dispute the unhelpful belief B	The new more effective belief I adopt to replace B, which leads to a different C in response to A.
Ex: My boss yelled at me today in front of my coworkers.	He has no right to embarrass me. It's not fair. I can't stand this.	I'm really mad and I want a drink.	Does my boss only yell at me? Is life always fair? Can I stand this without a drink?	My boss yells at everyone sooner or later. Life isn't fair. That didn't feel great, and it's over. My boss isn't worth giving up my long-term goals.

Tool 5.3: Practice problem solving

Date:

Use this Tool to explore how you might solve a large or small problem. Refer to the five-step problem-solving guide on page 63.

What is the root of the problem?

How could I address the problem?

Idea:	**Likeliness to work (0-10):**
1.	1.
2.	2.
3.	3.
4.	4.
5.	5.

Which idea will I try?

What individual steps should I take as part of my plan? You can also refer to Tool 3.3, the change-plan worksheet, on page 30.

Tool 5.3: Practice problem solving

Date:	
Use this Tool to explore how you might solve a large or small problem. Refer to the five-step problem-solving guide on page 63.	
What is the root of the problem?	
How could I address the problem?	
Idea: 1. 2. 3. 4. 5.	**Likeliness to work (0-10):** 1. 2. 3. 4. 5.
Which idea will I try?	
What individual steps should I take as part of my plan? You can also refer to Tool 3.3, the change-plan worksheet, on page 30.	

Tool 5.3: Practice problem solving

Date:	
Use this Tool to explore how you might solve a large or small problem. Refer to the five-step problem-solving guide on page 63.	
What is the root of the problem?	
How could I address the problem?	
Idea: 1. 2. 3. 4. 5.	**Likeliness to work (0-10):** 1. 2. 3. 4. 5.
Which idea will I try?	
What individual steps should I take as part of my plan? You can also refer to Tool 3.3, the change-plan worksheet, on page 30.	

Tool 5.5: Setting healthy boundaries

You can build confidence by communicating small boundaries before you broach big ones. What small boundaries can you begin setting? It's a good idea to practice on people in your life who aren't closest to you, too.

What small boundaries would you like to communicate?

Who	What	How
Ex: Colleague	Wash own coffee mugs	I feel frustrated when you don't wash your own coffee mug. Can I ask you to please start doing that?

What larger boundaries might you want to communicate with some practice?

Who	What	How

Tool 5.5: Setting healthy boundaries

You can build confidence by communicating small boundaries before you broach big ones. What small boundaries can you begin setting? It's a good idea to practice on people in your life who aren't closest to you, too.

What small boundaries would you like to communicate?

Who	What	How
Ex: Colleague	Wash own coffee mugs	I feel frustrated when you don't wash your own coffee mug. Can I ask you to please start doing that?

What larger boundaries might you want to communicate with some practice?

Who	What	How

Tool 5.5: Setting healthy boundaries

You can build confidence by communicating small boundaries before you broach big ones. What small boundaries can you begin setting? It's a good idea to practice on people in your life who aren't closest to you, too.

What small boundaries would you like to communicate?

Who	What	How
Ex: Colleague	Wash own coffee mugs	I feel frustrated when you don't wash your own coffee mug. Can I ask you to please start doing that?

What larger boundaries might you want to communicate with some practice?

Who	What	How

Tool 6.1: Check your lifestyle balance (lifestyle balance wheel[4])

Date:

Each spoke of the wheel represents an area of your life. Examples include family, friends, spirituality, romance, health, career, and finances. Some of your values (page 29) might also appear.

Rate your satisfaction (not how much energy you spend) in each aspect of your life by putting a dot on the center line. The outside edge is totally satisfied, while the inner corner is totally unsatisfied. Then connect the dots and see what shape you get. The rounder the wheel, the more balanced your life is.

See an example and tips on the next pages.

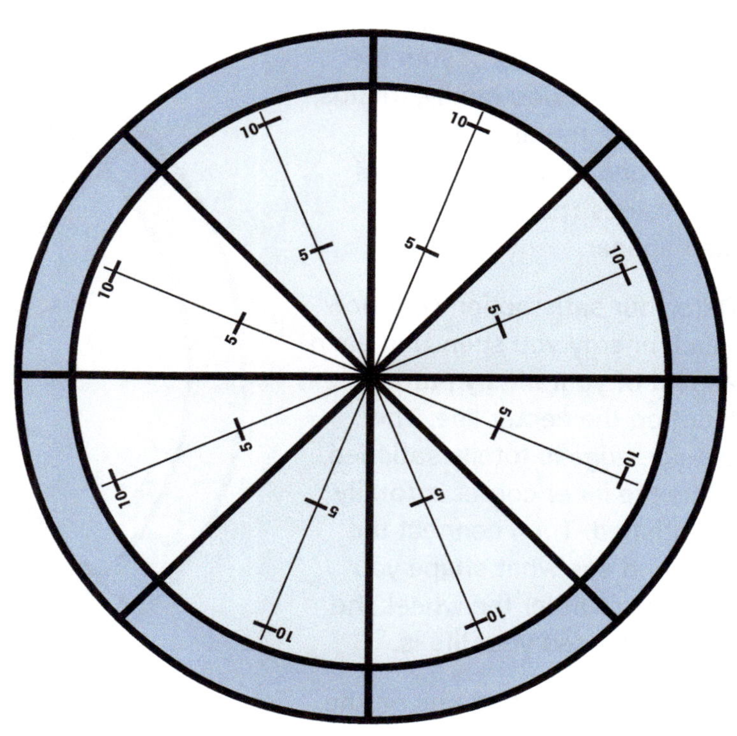

Highest-scoring categories	Lowest-scoring categories
1	8
2	7
3	6
4	5

Ask yourself:

- Would this wheel roll?
- What areas need more or less attention?
- How well does my wheel reflect my values?
- Am I involved in too much?
- How much time do I spend caring for others? For myself?

Notes and plans:

Tool 6.1: Check your lifestyle balance (lifestyle balance wheel[4])

Date:

Each spoke of the wheel represents an area of your life. Examples include family, friends, spirituality, romance, health, career, and finances. Some of your values (page 29) might also appear.

Rate your satisfaction (not how much energy you spend) in each aspect of your life by putting a dot on the center line. The outside edge is totally satisfied, while the inner corner is totally unsatisfied. Then connect the dots and see what shape you get. The rounder the wheel, the more balanced your life is.

See an example and tips on the next pages.

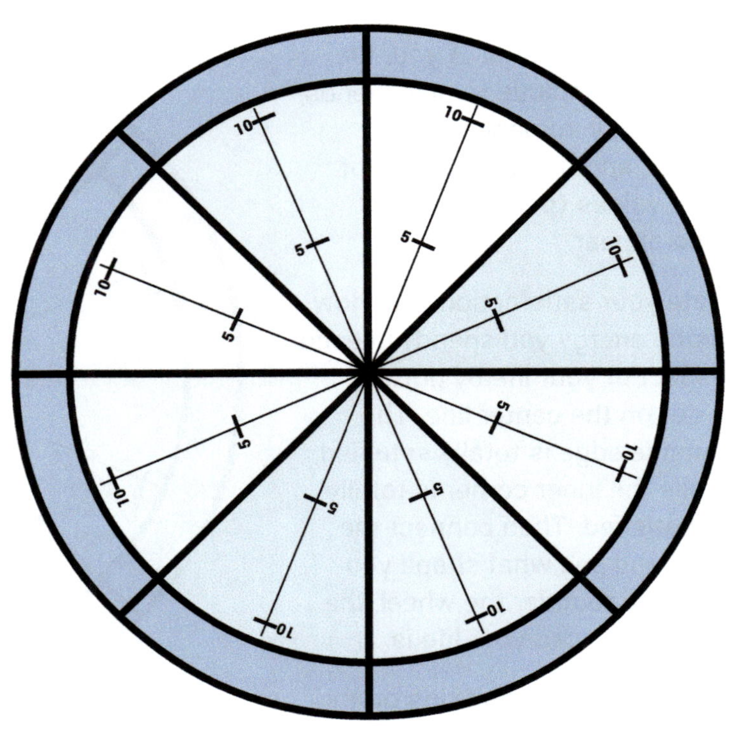

Highest-scoring categories	Lowest-scoring categories
1	8
2	7
3	6
4	5

Ask yourself:	**Notes and plans:**
• Would this wheel roll? • What areas need more or less attention? • How well does my wheel reflect my values? • Am I involved in too much? • How much time do I spend caring for others? For myself?	

Tool 6.1: Check your lifestyle balance (lifestyle balance wheel[4])

Date:

Each spoke of the wheel represents an area of your life. Examples include family, friends, spirituality, romance, health, career, and finances. Some of your values (page 29) might also appear.

Rate your satisfaction (not how much energy you spend) in each aspect of your life by putting a dot on the center line. The outside edge is totally satisfied, while the inner corner is totally unsatisfied. Then connect the dots and see what shape you get. The rounder the wheel, the more balanced your life is.

See an example and tips on the next pages.

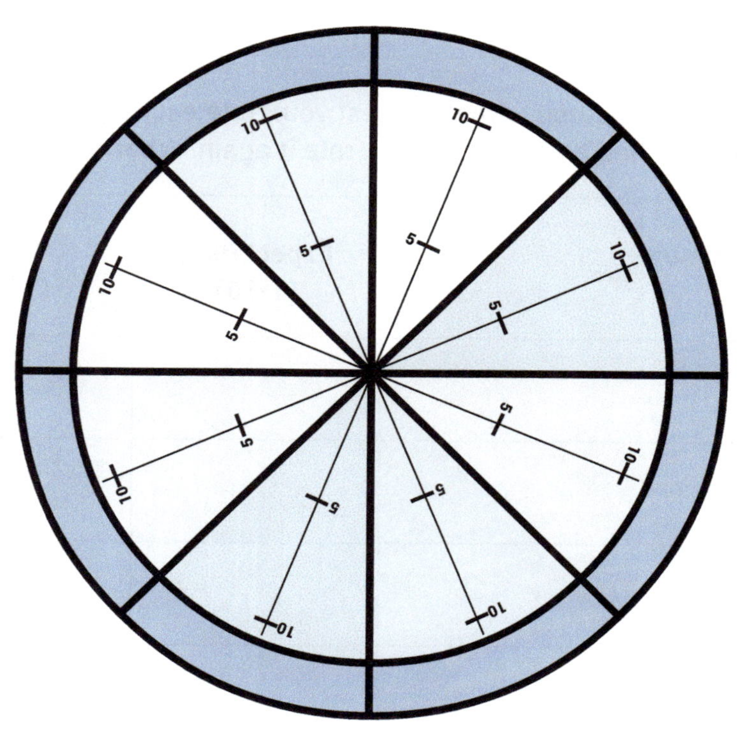

Highest-scoring categories	Lowest-scoring categories
1	8
2	7
3	6
4	5

Ask yourself:

- Would this wheel roll?
- What areas need more or less attention?
- How well does my wheel reflect my values?
- Am I involved in too much?
- How much time do I spend caring for others? For myself?

Notes and plans:

Tool 6.2: Explore new pursuits and passions

(vital absorbing creative interests)

Date:

Jot down pursuits that interest you. Rate each by how much you expect to enjoy it. Once you've had a chance to try it, rate it again. What surprises you?

Pursuit	**Expectation (1-10)**	**Reality (1-10)**	**Comments/thoughts**

Tool 6.2: Explore new pursuits and passions

(vital absorbing creative interests)

Date:

Jot down pursuits that interest you. Rate each by how much you expect to enjoy it. Once you've had a chance to try it, rate it again. What surprises you?

Pursuit	**Expectation (1-10)**	**Reality (1-10)**	**Comments/thoughts**

Tool 6.2: Explore new pursuits and passions

(vital absorbing creative interests)

Date:

Jot down pursuits that interest you. Rate each by how much you expect to enjoy it. Once you've had a chance to try it, rate it again. What surprises you?

Pursuit	**Expectation (1-10)**	**Reality (1-10)**	**Comments/thoughts**

Tool 6.3: Set an effective goal

Goal:

Specific	Measurable	Agreeable	Realistic	Time-bound

Tasks to reach my goal:

Tool 6.3: Set an effective goal

Goal:

Specific	Measurable	Agreeable	Realistic	Time-bound

Tasks to reach my goal:

Tool 6.3: Set an effective goal

Goal:

Specific	Measurable	Agreeable	Realistic	Time-bound

Tasks to reach my goal:

Tool 6.3: Set an effective goal

Goal:

Specific	Measurable	Agreeable	Realistic	Time-bound

Tasks to reach my goal:

Tool 6.3: Set an effective goal

Goal:

Specific	Measurable	Agreeable	Realistic	Time-bound

Tasks to reach my goal: